Grow Young Without Plastic Surgery

JOHN JAMES BELMAR

belmarjh@caribsurf.com

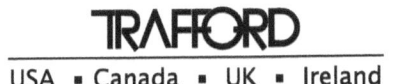

USA ▪ Canada ▪ UK ▪ Ireland

Note for Librarians: A cataloguing record for this book is available from Library and Archives Canada at www.collectionscanada.ca/amicus/index-e.html
ISBN 1-4120-9429-1

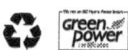

Printed on paper with minimum 30% recycled fibre.
Trafford's print shop runs on "green energy" from solar, wind and other environmentally-friendly power sources.

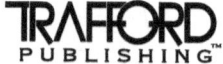

Offices in Canada, USA, Ireland and UK

Book sales for North America and international:
Trafford Publishing, 6E–2333 Government St.,
Victoria, BC V8T 4P4 CANADA
phone 250 383 6864 (toll-free 1 888 232 4444)
fax 250 383 6804; email to orders@trafford.com
Book sales in Europe:
Trafford Publishing (UK) Limited, 9 Park End Street, 2nd Floor
Oxford, UK OX1 1HH UNITED KINGDOM
phone 44 (0)1865 722 113 (local rate 0845 230 9601)
facsimile 44 (0)1865 722 868; info.uk@trafford.com
Order online at:
trafford.com/06-1184

10 9 8 7 6 5 4 3

Acknowledgements

I must first acknowledge that I am blessed by the Creator, and destiny has led me through many intuitive and spiritual awakenings, through which I received understanding to fulfill this assignment. I am extremely grateful for the opportunity to fulfill my part in this honorable service of leading you as a people to a higher level of self-consciousness.

Through the years I have been secretly practicing the understanding of rejuvenation which is revealed to me through dreams and visions.

My physical rejuvenation began to become obvious about ten years ago. My critical Uncle Sam said to me, "Everyone is getting old beside my nephew." I asked, "Who is this nephew you are talking about?" He replied, "Look at yourself in the mirror. I am your uncle. I knew when you were born."

The number of persons who have been questioning my physical appearance of rejuvenation is astounding. My cousin Leon Tomson, who is closer to me than a brother, inquired of me, "No one is able to do what you are doing. You are not getting old. What is the secret?"

The title of this book came to me because of a conversation with the manager and exercise instructor of a gym where I accompanied my grand daughter, Deka to be enrolled; it was my gift to her. When I presented my drivers license and a credit card, he looked at the documents and asked, "Is this your credit card? You could not be this old." "Yes I am!" "So what is your secret?" he asked, "Are you on a special diet? Do you exercise? Have you done plastic surgery?"

The many persons who have been asking questions about my appearance are too many to mention their names. I therefore extend my sincere gratitude to them as a group for the confidence and motivation that goad me because their questions have inspired me and made me realize that the time has come to share this knowledge with the world. Notwithstanding, there are other persons with whom I am more closely acquainted and must say to them a personal thank you, for their help and motivation.

Ms. Verile Ann Jones, my devoted editor who is the most generous and loving person I have ever known. From the first day we met she has been an inspiration.

Thanks to my cousin, Leon Tomson who has been a brother in spirit. I recognized how controversial a questioning mind you possess. Your judgment and inspiration I deeply appreciate. Thank you!

Susan Tomson, my cousin, friend and student who has been very supportive in my quest for knowledge, with whom I felt comfortable to discuss the many challenges that I had to overcome. You are worthy of praise.

Mr. Kyron Barker, my friend and neighbor who is a brilliant university graduate. Thanks very much for your proof reading skills my friend!

Dr. Michael Howard, Professor in Economics at the University of the West Indies. Thanks, my friend for your critical assessment of the script. Your comments and assessment were well taken.

Special thanks for Mr. Rawle Culbard for the cover photographs he took.

Foreword

The information outlined in this book contains carefully arranged affirmations to help the Mind delete many religious dogmas and mythical beliefs, so as to accept the priceless divine truths based on a comprehensive biblical research of the New Testament. The concepts are true, but to most of us they are unprecedented even though the functions of Nature's abundant supply demonstrate compelling evidence.

This book is simply presented so that it would be of benefit to all.

Some of the challenging words used and their meaning are listed on Pages (*xvii*) to (*xxiv*) at the back for your convenience if necessary.

Introduction

I am seventy-five years young and an example of a rejuvenated person. Many years ago, and to present, my relatives, friends, acquaintances and associates have been inquiring as to the secrets of my youthful appearance.

This book reveals some of these secrets about:

- The natural ways to rejuvenate without the use of drugs.

- Understanding the functions of emotion which triggers rejuvenation

- How important is emotion (*ebullience*) to positive affirmations.

- How the beauty and abundance of Mother Nature to supply is intended to enrich the soul and bring opulence into your life.

- Understanding why every thought is a powerful prayer in motion.

- Discovering that the body is a spiritual temple that is not designed to age, but rejuvenate because of the thought process and its physiological functions that induce emotion.

- Understanding the hidden powers of the mind and the discipline of emotion that will lead to prosperity.

- Understanding that there is a difference between the soul and the spirit. This knowledge and understanding leads to a high level of self esteem and increases wholeness of mind and body.

Aging is a mental stigma, and I have discovered how to obliterate it. I have discovered how to stay young by removing the stigma of aging from the subconscious mind, so that rejuvenation can take effect.

The book reveals personal benefits of praying for one's enemies. How and why our emotions attract to us the unwanted conditions we wish to avoid. In addition, it provides knowledge on how to obliterate the emotions of fear, hate, greed and deceptions that cause self-destruction.

The book is about the psychology of aging and the knowledge of how to rejuvenate through a *specific type of meditation* where you protract and assimilate the flux of Mother Nature that enriches the soul. This experience can transform you into a magnetic force that will enrich your lives with peace, love, happiness and prosperity.

Table of Contents

1

THE TRUE BEAUTY OF SELF

Emotion is the spiritual force that transforms our imaginations into experiences. Hence, ethereal ideas induce emotion that will cause rejuvenation. Why not create imaginations of youth, health, love, peace, beauty, and opulence?

At the age of eleven, my attention was captivated by a tender grass plant which was protruding through the hard surface of stone and pitch in order to absorb air, sunlight and water, which are vital for the plant to grow to express beauty and purpose. I wondered, if there was an invisible, omnipresent, all-knowing someone, or something, which provided the sustenance that produces and sustains the proper temperature, sunlight, water, and oxygen that every life form needs to survive! And what is my purpose here {on Earth} in this space and time, that all these things are provided for my survival?

Through the years from a child I have grown to become a fully developed adult. I am now seventy five years young. Yes, I am young because everywhere I go, whether on business or pleasure, people want to know the secret of my youthful appearance; especially those who have known me for several years.

The secret of my youth is accredited to my understanding of the nature of the thought process. You too can rejuvenate as I have been doing over the past twenty years. However, before we get into the actual psychological application of rejuvenation, there are some simple, natural, innate truths that must be told about the self and the thought process.

Let us begin with three questions: [1] Why are you always thinking? [2] Do you always choose your thoughts, or most of the time do they just seem to invade your mind? [3] How often do you pray?

You have probably heard many people proclaim, "I do not believe in prayer." If you are one of those it is because you lack knowledge of your spiritual self and the power of your thoughts and emotion to manifest ideas into experiences.

The act of thinking is prayer. Do you know that every thought is a powerful prayer in motion? Yes, I am the evidence of that truth because in my mind, I am a young man, and my body expresses it.

Do you remember the comedian by the name of Flip Wilson? His favorite innuendo on stage was, "What you see is what you get!" What Flip Wilson was implying is that *what you see in your mind, is what you will get out of life.* Think about it for a moment. Then study this favorite quotation of mine, "consciousness produces life" Whatever you are conscious of will manifest into experiences. The following are a few of the questions I am being asked everyday by relatives, acquaintances, friends, and associates:

- Are you on a special diet?
  I'm not!

- Do you exercise?
  I take casual walks occasionally!

- Have you done plastic surgery?
  I have never considered it!

- Well, tell me, what's the secret?

The act of aging is a psychological condition caused by false beliefs. Every thought is a powerful prayer in motion. It is being said, that, you are, what you eat! It is also true to say that, you are the product of your thoughts! One cannot stop the thought process therefore; you are continuously engaged in the act of prayer. Prayer is a natural phenomenon, but the majority of us do not understand the ramifications of the quality of thoughts we are entertaining. We are continuously praying for one thing or another. Simply by thinking, whether we are in church, sitting at home, walking or driving a car; we are using the power of prayer. Without such awareness, we become victims of ignorance.

Many people fail to realize the things they desire in life. The truth is, their desires are not what they entertain in thoughts and feeling. Emotions are spiritual forces of attraction. Since you cannot stop thinking, are you not curious to know how your thoughts affect your life? Negative emotions attract unpleasant experiences. They also generate and transmit magnetic vibrations of their nature which attract even more experiences of the quality of your thoughts.

While many persons entertain thoughts of greed, envy, hate, and deception, they expect peace, love, success, joy, and happiness to be in their lives, but the principles that govern the thought process will not allow it. Every function in the Universe is governed by one or many principles, with no exception to our thoughts.

You can only reap 'fruits' [things] from the kinds of 'seeds' which you plant in the Earth. So too, you will harvest only the things of your thoughts and ideas which your character expresses. That which your character expresses is what you are within, and what you become within your *soul* shall manifest itself into flesh. You judge people's ages by their appearance; when they do not match the conviction within your subconscious mind, you will ask why not?

It is crucial that you develop a comprehensive understanding of how your mind with its unlimited powers works. Thoughts unleash the unlimited powers of your mind. Your physiological functions are in collaboration with mind and body to bring into your life, experiences of joy and a constant high on ethereal ideas. But because of ignorance of the power of thoughts, and in desperation to obtain such fulfillment from the natural beauty of Nature which is ubiquitous, many persons experiment with deleterious drugs to satisfy a spiritual need. Such actions ultimately destroy the body and deprive it of a natural function that is spiritual in nature.

In your world of imagination you must ask of the spirit of life within you, to fill your mind, your soul, and your body with the spirit of eternal bliss: peace, love, health, youth, beauty, and abundance. All of which Mother Nature's creative activities are constantly expressing. When last have you been to the botanical garden to observe the beauty of the trees in the fall, and admire the constant change and beauty of the clouds? We were not made to live only by physical substance; for bread shall only satisfy the stomach, the mind needs to be fed also.

The rejuvenation of soul and body is a psychological process, but a nutritious diet helps the process of rejuvenation.

When you are disciplined to a healthy nutritious diet the body will become more receptive, and in tune with ideas of divine qualities that produce spiritual self-awareness and rejuvenation.

The process of aging and rejuvenation is mental and psychological and must be treated as such. It is well known that, *every cause originate in the mind.* A condition that manifests in the mind, which can transform the soul and body accordingly, is independent of nutritious diet and therefore must be treated psychologically.

To become whole both in mind and body, we need emotional substance as well. Make a daily habit to give love and attention to the natural things of Nature, and she shall *reciprocate* to you her energy of beauty and power.

The many subconscious images, like the

negatives of film by which you compare other people's appearances, will affect the condition of your soul. As age progresses your soul gradually transforms, as it takes the wizened resemblance of your convictions of the aging process. The body is but only a mirror reflection of your soul; hence by a principle of thought law, your physical form must progressively transform to outwardly express the conviction you have ignorantly accepted and impressed on the soul.

The nature of the spirit is quite different from the soul. By influence of the conscious mind in collaboration with the subconscious mind, changes to the soul are enforced. The spirit however, never changes. It maintains the original most beautiful form of God's creation since the original Adam was created. Can you imagine the immaculate beauty of your spirit?

Consider this analogy: The seed of the fruit holds the unchangeable pattern of the tree and its fruits and therefore cannot be altered. The spirit of man is the divine image of God's self that God created in His image and likeness. Whereas the soul of man took form the moment that man form the personal concept of "himself" as a physical being. That was the genesis of his soul. The soul is continuously changing in accord with man's conscious experiences. The body occasionally changes to express the joy or sorrow of the soul.

Heaven is a state of mind: a state of spiritual consciousness. Nevertheless it is as real as the dimension of earth's reality. The consciousness of that state Adam lost when he took on the physical form of flesh. He became so mundane, that he drifted away from that mental condition which is the true home of the soul, where the soul and spirit shall forever reside in spiritual opulence.

Until such time as you achieve knowledge of the spiritual source of beauty and opulence, the transformation of your soul to equal the beauty of your spirit will not be achieved. As you forge your way to progressively achieve perfection of the soul, it becomes equal to that of the spirit. We grow by way of the negative experiences we suffer through ignorance of who we are and where we belong.

When you are in love you take on a luminous glow, and your friends and acquaintances will ask what is going on in your life! Conversely, when you are in a bad mood they are likely to keep their distance. Is this not evidence that your body is a mirror image of your soul's experiences?

You are the sole product of your thoughts and emotions. This is why the master teacher in the Holy Bible advises us on emotional discipline.

In Matthew 5:41, "And whosoever shall compel thee to go a mile, go with him twain." In Matthew 5:44-45, "Love your enemies, bless them that curse you, do good to them that hate you, and pray for them which despitefully use you, and persecute you."

This advice is in direct collaboration with the principles of our thought process. Why should I acquiesce to such manipulations if not to refrain from anger? You should avoid irate persons. They are deleterious to your health, peace, prosperity, and happiness. Your physiological functions are the *ad hoc* by which the flux of Nature expresses its Divine purpose in you.

13

I cannot continue this work if I refrain from giving due credit to the source of all my information. In my view Jesus is the greatest teacher on the subject of positive thinking. I am blessed with a gift to understand the principles he lived and taught. The understanding and practice of which I am rejuvenating, therefore I shall refer to his work occasionally. One cannot say that he or she is positive and not characterize such optimism. Jesus' life exemplified the character he was as a man.

As you study the contents of the following chapter, you must realize that every form of human suffering came about because of disobedience of the principles Jesus presented. Bring your thoughts in harmony with the divine examples of Nature's beauty, opulence, and love in which nature is supplying sustenance to all the living things and creatures that

She created, and that shall be the end of hardship and suffering.

Notepad

_____

_____

_____

_____

_____

_____

_____

_____

_____

_____

_____

_____

_____

_____

_____

_____

_____

_____

_____

_____

2

CONVERSANT WITH INVISIBLE REALITY

If you do not have any previous knowledge of this subject, your present state of awareness will only allow your senses to experience a *limited amount* of the material things and actions of Earth's reality. There is an invisible dimension from which the things of Earth manifest and materialize.

The things of Earth cause deceptive delusions to your senses and deprive you of benefits of a higher form of existence. Nevertheless, by observing Nature's actions through her physical forms, will enable you to see past the delusions which the appearances of physical things create. Conversely, the things of nature are also designed to serve as examples and teaching tools that will take you into the inner or invisible reality of greater peace, love, beauty, and opulence. The flux of nature is a paradigm of divine principles.

The following practice of abstract reasoning is designed to take you into a much higher state of reality - the place of infinite supply, and provide you with knowledge to access and benefit from the invisible source from where you can add supply to your life experiences.

I will reiterate many of the nebulous journeys and examples so that you will not lose your way on this invisible road to the source that created you. The experience is like going back home to where you belong. Bear in mind that you too are invisible in a visible body of flesh. You are about to embark on an intuitive journey. The use of all your senses is required if you are to arrive home safely without delay.

Although you have eyes, because of the delusions of material things you are not able to see and feel the unbreakable union between you and the source of life, and the process by which it is accessible. You must become a positive magnet of attraction by constructive application of your thoughts.

Recognize that ideas and thoughts are invisible entities and that awareness induces emotion which becomes the evidence of whatsoever you accept as reality. Understand that whenever you allow saturation of any emotional quality to invade your mind, the substance of those things will attract similar experiences into your life. Those experiences, if they are unpleasant will be the punishment you will bear for wrongfully applying the power of your thoughts.

The following is one of much exercise that can spontaneously increase self consciousness. Because of this experience you will realize that the good things that were only wishful thoughts are now a spiritual reality that you can manifest in your life. This source that rejuvenates youth and healing could also provide your other desires. It is the spiritual source from which all things evolved.

In addition to rejuvenation of youth and healing, the source of life could be considered to be the only true panacea.

Allow me to be your docent in your discovery of self:

1. Ruminate the following. One usually says *"Food for thought!"* Be still, and observe that the source that created the things of Nature for the sustenance of the human race has projected you out of itself into this wealth it has created. Use your imagination and observe the affects of the Sun on the Sea; the rain showers to Earth produce vegetation, water and oxygen to sustain life, and the beauty of Nature that induces *ebullience* to enrich the soul. All of which is for your comfort and pleasure. Therefore, you are an inheritor to all things that have been created for your existence. You are the reason why the universe is. Practice this exercise daily to develop your sense of inheritance.

2. Observe that there is an invisible presence seeking to express itself through you by way of ideas and thoughts. We receive ideas. We do not create them!

Sit pensively under a tree, by a lake or river if possible and endeavor to feel a sense of oneness with the environment. The breath of life connects you to all things in the universe. The only thing that can separate you from this beauty and opulence that is yours by nature is hate, jealousy, and greed. The above practice will give you an awareness of oneness with the universal opulence.

3. As you observe and analyze this price-less truth, be aware of the ever chang-ing beauty of the clouds and twitter-ing music of beautifully contrasting colorful feathers of the birds on the branches of trees. They are all supplies intended to induce ebullience. We live, move, and have our being in it. We are made of it, and belong to it. You must therefore establish a parent and child relationship with it. This is why Jesus proclaimed "The Father and I are

one." You must forge your way to become one with the source of Nature's supply. For what you have become in spirit it shall manifest itself in your life experiences.

To protect yourself from negative emotions you must forgive your enemies and love them. That seems not realistic by society's standard but that is the principle of your spiritual nature: live by the law or suffer the consequences. Whatever thought vibrations you send to others they shall ultimately return to you and you will receive the pleasure or pain of their influence.

At this point in your journey for truth we have observed many of the basic principles that will prepare you for soul and body rejuvenation. There are others like me who have obtained this level of self consciousness, but choose to live in an environment away from public view for various reasons.

Allow me to use an analogy of a library with hundreds of basement floors. The floor above road surface is your conscious mind, and the floors below zero level should be considered dimensions of the subconscious mind. In every reincarnated life that you return to Earth another subconscious floor takes form. So, can you imagine the myriad depth of your subconscious mind? Can you comprehend the prodigious volumes of the stigma of aging ingrained in that phase of your mind?

The stigma of aging is simple to understand. Whenever you converse with anyone, and on many occasions it happened to me, because the question of revealing your age is not evasive in our society. The persons that interviewed me in the preceding five years suddenly became inter-rogators, by asking how old I am even when they have my documents in front of them.

At times they will compliment me by say-ing "You look well for your age. Gosh, I wish I could look like you when I become your age. Do you take plastic surgery? Are you on a special diet? What kind of exercise you do?" On one occasion my friend's daughter looked at me with a curious expression. When her mother inquired into the reason, her daughter's response was, "He looks younger than the last time I saw him." It has become an everyday experience for me, and that was when I decided it was time to pro-duce this book.

The people who are questioning my ap-pearance, judge me by comparing my ap-pearance to their own expectations of the aging process that are engraved in their subconscious minds. Those imprints are stored like that of the negatives of a camera. When you reveal your age to anyone the person will subconsciously compare your information and appearance to the negatives with their conviction of how you should look, for the age you revealed.

When the information you give does not match their expectation they will challenge you. So each person's physical form, (because of thought principle), must progressively age to become the negative beliefs of his/her soul. The soul of each individual becomes the pattern of his or her expectation of others. Since the body is a mirror of the soul you should understand why the process continues endlessly. To stop the aging process and start rejuvenation the subconscious imprints must be obliterated from the subconscious mind of the one who desires to rejuvenate. How was I able to accomplish that?

To successfully rejuvenate your mind and body, you must pensively ruminate on the beauty and abundance of Nature's supply to experience an inseparable union with the flux of Nature's beauty and opulence, to the point of inclusive conviction that the Universe is because of you.

You can eliminate the darkness from a room by the activation of a light switch. So too, concepts of the universality of things shall replace the stigma of limitation.

At this juncture in our discussion you should realize that the body is but only a mirror reflection of your soul's experiences. You must therefore, refrain from judging others by appearance. Be aware that the power of each individual's belief (the magic of your mind) will manifest itself. The magic of your mind shall produce the *physical illusion* that expresses your conviction of aging, whether or not your beliefs are in accord with spiritual truth.

At this point have you not come to recognize the power of thoughts? Use your imagination and create a new mental image of yourself; one of youth, health, and beauty. Since the subconscious mind accepts every *emotional* suggestion as an already existing truth, the mind will delete the old-age negatives and replace them with your new conviction of youth. The process is psychological and subconscious. All that is required of you is to make your new self image part of your *daily consciousness*. As you walk the streets, silently affirm "I am becoming youthful, healthy, and happy!" Do this as often as possible and nature will produce the result. If you faithfully apply these exercises secretly, after a period of about thirty days your friends and acquaintances will approach you with complementary statements about your appearance. Look not for the results; others will bring them to your attention.

Notepad

3

PHYSICAL REJUVENATION

This chapter provides insight into the functions of your conscious mind and the wisdom to understand and become acquainted with its creative powers. This is mandatory so that you can subjugate its creative energies.

The learning process of self-awareness is not abstruse but nurturing. As you progress, you will realize that mind teaches itself. Most of us have the notion that Nature's method is so dissembled that one cannot discover one's self by observing her ways. The converse is obviously protuberant. If you give love and attention to the things that Nature produces they will reveal their secrets to you. The experience could be salubrious.

There are several levels of consciousness but in this Earth dimension we only require the use of four. The majority of us consciously use only two. Herein we shall observe the three levels most frequently used.

1. The Physical Consciousness: This phase makes you conscious of your physical being and the immediate environment.

2. The Subjective Consciousness: This phase allows you to apply reason and logic to judge whether or not an experience is pragmatic or deceptive. The functions of the subjective mind are like that of a security guard. When an idea or suggestion attempts to pass the

subjective mind to gain approval in the subconscious mind, the idea or suggestion has to convince the subjective guard that it is a genuine experience of the conscious mind, not just an idea or a suggestion. If the subjective guard is not convinced that the idea or suggestion is a genuine experience of the conscious mind, they will be blocked from entering into the subconscious mind because they lack sufficient *emotional substance* (faith) to convince the subjective mind that they are true experiences of the Conscious mind.

3. Subconscious: This phase is the storehouse of memories. With or without any effort of yours, it records all experiences, and reproduces those which contain strong emotional desires. You need to develop a character that will recognize the benefits derived from the actions of the subconscious mind.

I again reiterate that the subconscious mind is the library within you which stores all your experiences, and has power to obviate or delete the unaccepted unpleasant experiences. If the conscious mind experiences a new reality, the subjective mind must approve that it is genuine before acceptance is granted. Mental reality of ideas and suggestions must contain strong *emotional desire* to pass through the subjective mind on its way into the subconscious mind. Hence, you should understand the quotation: "Be it unto you according to your belief." I aver that the three phases of mind, namely: conscious, subjective, and subconscious, are designed to bring you the finest things in life.

The subconscious is that phase of your mind that brings into physical manifestation experiences of the things you believe as true or possible. You will have to become acquainted with your subconscious mind through meditation. Your subconscious self is the genius within you.

The majority of us are ignorant of this all powerful self within. Are you aware that you are the same in substance like the creator? We are made by him and are of him! We therefore inherit some degree of his creative powers.

Be aware that consciousness is not a physical function which perishes with the body in death. You must realize that the five senses form an outer expression of the consciousness within. And that the soul is an ever changing form of self. When you use the power of suggestion, and images of imagination to influence the conscious mind; only if the imagination produces *emotion* will it impress the subjective mind that the imagination is a reality of the conscious mind so that it is allowed to continue its journey into the subconscious mind, the source in which it shall manifest itself into an experience that you must accept thereafter. Subsequently, the subjective mind allows whatsoever the *conscious* mind believes, to enter into the *subconscious* mind. Whatever the conscious mind accepts, will enter the subconscious mind. Whatever suggestion or image is allowed in the subconscious mind, will influence change in the *soul*. Whatever directive the soul receives from the subconscious mind, the soul then transforms to become that new image that is forced upon it by the subconscious mind. Since the body is but a mirror of the soul, the body takes upon itself that recent transformation to express the new image of the soul. As a result, you will experience physical rejuvenation or the converse.

One's consciousness of self begins to

change at the age of an infant and unfolds in cycles of seven years through the continuous process of self development. Through the developing process, a child of fourteen is unlike one of seven years. When one becomes twenty one years, his or her conviction and attitude about life is not the same as when he or she was fourteen. Consciousness is a continuous unfolding process that makes us individually different according to the state of awareness in which we are functioning at any given time in our development.

As one moves through life from one level of consciousness to another, one perceives things differently. Even some of us who are in the same age group are not exactly alike, because individually, we are possessed with aptitudes which we subconsciously developed in previous lives' experiences.

As one's creative nature unfolds into self-awareness, one's physical form will be transformed and will illuminate his or her state of awareness. The evidence of such transformation becomes the truth that will goad others to follow in search of peace, health, rejuvenation, ebullience and prosperity. My ability to rejuvenate is an example of that.

At the moment of death, the entity within, leaves the body (a consciousness that most of us believe is only physical), but will surprisingly experience he/she is still alive without a body (at the moment of death) because the soul and spirit is immortal. At this time you are very much alive, but invisible to those around you.

Everything goes through a transition not observed by the majority. With man, male and female, ours begin at birth and proceeds in death to eternity. True, life is eternal and omnipresent. The hereafter is an ongoing conscious and subconscious journey.

How convenient for most of us to believe that life ends at the moment of death. Such a concept gives one the green light to deceive others. The false belief that there is only one life and that there is no ramification to pay for unjust deeds!

This way of thinking is convenient for those who refuse to accept responsibility for their deceptive behavior. They are blind to the fact that everything is governed by a principle of divine justice or remuneration. As we give, we receive. Certainly, "What goes around comes around." One must pay or reap just reward for one's thoughts and actions.

By now you should realize that this unfolding knowledge of self-development provides wisdom which enables you to achieve more than rejuvenation, and there are prices to be paid. Emotional *discipline* stands out to be the most demanding one of them. To help refresh your understanding, I shall reiterate from time to time.

To develop self-esteem, and become a magnet to the things which you have always dreamed of having, you must bring your thoughts in harmony with the ways of Nature, how she creates and distributes indiscriminately. You must think and feel you are one with her energies of beauty and opulence. We are made from those same spiritual energies which are producing our supplies. Before there was anything, there was God, and everything is made by Him, and is of Him! All things in the universe originated from one source of energy.

Since a conviction in thought expresses itself by emotion, it stands to reason that *emotion* is the evidence of the things of your *thoughts*, or the evidence of things hoped for.

You should *scrupulously* control your feelings, so that it shall not ever transform unpleasant thoughts into emotions of fear, hate, envy, greed, etcetera, or else we shall be fully occupied with unpleasant manifold experiences.

The above reveals that emotional substance is necessary to induce manifestation: How easily we supply negative emotions to anger and hate? Without positive emotional substance your efforts will be without merit. Here again, I must reiterate the importance of the exercise of *abstract inductive reasoning*. This practice of induction induces physiological inductive energies that shall make you consciously united with the energies of the creative spirit. It provides knowledge, conviction, wisdom, and understanding that shall enable you to take vigorous control of your thoughts.

Induce emotion only when necessary for you to create that which is good. It is imperative that you frequently practice the exercise of induction daily.

If you are unable to induce emotion into your favorable imagination your desire cannot manifest itself. I must again reiterate; *emotion* is the substance that *gives life to your imagination.* And the practice of inductive reasoning will saturate you in Nature's flux as it takes you into a higher level of oneness with Nature's plethora. When you become enriched with nature's wealth, you will be a positive magnet of attraction.

The emotional substance of wealth you have become shall attract the material things of your feelings. *Without* achieving the *consciousness* that you are one with the energy of spiritual supply the subconscious mind cannot command material wealth to materialize for you. Therefore you must scrupulously guard the power of your *consciousness* and *emotion,* and use them only to manifest positive desires.

Notepad

4

CHOICE OF EMOTION

Never get emotional when negative ideas invade your thoughts. They sneak into your consciousness and before you realize it, emotion of hate, greed, fear, and deception manifest themselves. The magnetic energies of the above emotions spontaneously detach you from your energies of health, youth, peace, love, and beauty. Hence, you should be prudent; be alert for those unwelcome intruders and delete them from your thoughts.

When you consciously choose a pleasant experience of the past, the unpleasant radicals will disappear from your mind.

Take this simple analogy for example; you turn on a light switch and the darkness disappears from your room. Your pleasant memories and positive imaginations are "switches" available to you. The memory of love is the best "switch"! Negative radicals must be subjugated if you are to enjoy true success, inner peace, health, joy, and happiness by constantly switching on the emotional lights when negative forces try to intervene.

If you were to look within yourself and observe your thoughts and feelings you will experience evidence of this truth. Such discipline shall endow you with power of self-control. You will come to realize that you are truly a temple of the creative spirit within. Pleasant thoughts will attract a plethora of beauty in your affairs. The practice of thought discipline is mandatory if you desire to *protract and assimilate* emotional energy of your desire from nature's bountiful supply.

PRACTICE:

Be quiescent and observe. Take into account the flux of Mother Nature's plethoric beauty. Her didactics of our spiritual nature is exemplary. Observe how her paradigm challenges you to take notice of the ways she produces abundance. They are constantly appealing for your attention to establish continuum with your physiological functions (the coordination of body and mind in harmony) to induce ebullience that will transform spiritual truth into material manifestation.

As you experience conviction with Nature's replete and your physiological functions that induce feelings, observe how both actions are in harmony to produce manifestation. Your mind must conceive this salient truth. It is an awareness that is necessary to establish a closer relationship with spiritual abundance, so practice the following exercise to sharpen your insight.

Take a walk and see how refreshing it feels to enjoy the beauty of Nature. Now make an effort to appreciate the things of nature's beauty that the eyes behold, and think of the process in motion that is influencing this because it is the function between body and mind that is producing feeling of ebullience and contentment that you are experiencing. The body and mind together are harmoniously engaged to produce a physiological effect which results in the manifestation of ebullience. That ebullience shall transform your facial expression. Especially if you can see in your mind's eye the process that is causing the transformation. When you are in the flux of Nature's Beauty and Abundance, see yourself as young, healthy and rich.

You must habitually observe the continuum between your body and the flux of Nature's profuseness. Subsequently, you within the body can claim inheritance of all that Nature produces and become mentally rich. Thereafter the law of attraction will bring into your life the experiences of your conscious mind.

The creator has not only provided material substance for our physical well-being, but has also provided spiritual supply by the same action of Nature's ever changing beauty. The physiological coordination of mind and body which induces renaissance is the *ad hoc* for receiving spiritual supply as well. Observe, although the body is physical, it is also designed to absorb and induce physiological effects that transform your physical appearance whereby rejuvenation becomes practical.

Continuous convictions of ethereal truth can transform the body to spirit.

Notepad

_____

_____

_____

_____

_____

_____

_____

_____

_____

_____

_____

_____

_____

_____

_____

_____

_____

_____

5

꒕꒖

POSITIVE AFFIRMATION

The understanding and use of Positive Affirmation is essential in the application and development of a higher self-consciousness.

Affirmations are natural expressions people emotionally use to express their beliefs and disbeliefs occasionally when challenged by an optimist. For a pessimist to become an optimist, it is crucial that he or she must expound his or her horizon of self-awareness in spiritual development. This is accomplished by the study and practice of the prescribed intuitive observance of Nature's ongoing creative abundant supply that provides our sustenance, so as to become aware of your true purpose in the scheme of things, and conclude that the universe is because of us! The practice of induction into Nature's abundance will mentally put you into the source of spiritual supply. You can never be overly saturated with this supply. Affirmation is worthless if you are not filled with the energy of spiritual supply.

The following group of affirmations is divided into two parts. The first part begins with "I am spiritually rich," This group of affirmations is for the few people who are so developed spiritually that they can identify as one with Mother Nature and the universe. Like Jesus, when he proclaimed the Christ, affirmed "The Father and I are one!" Do you have any acceptable explanation to support that you, Mother Nature, and the Universe are one? If you come into that level of self awareness, you will also discover that you and the Father are also one. Then you earn the authority to proclaim that you are one with the Father.

The second group of affirmations is for those who have yet to grow into the above level of spiritual self-awareness. If you belong to the second group it will be productive to start your affirmation with "I choose," or "I desire." To keep increasing your conviction of self-awareness, pensively practice the intuitive observance of Nature's cycle of supply at least three times daily.

Written affirmations are more affective when the prints are so small that you are hardly conscious of its visibility substance. Subliminal suggestions are more influential on the Mind; so powerful it could be at times, it renders the subjective mind ineffective. The subjective Mind is that function of consciousness which determines whether an idea is true or false.

The following are affirmations that one may use in accord with his or her understanding, conviction, experience, and belief. The affirmation you choose must be in harmony with your *'feeling'* at the time of usage. For example if you are sick do not say "I am well" but instead say "I am being healed with every breath I take." Having understood the principle you may create your own affirmation or use any of the following:

GROUP ONE:

"I am spiritually rich!"

"I am spirit; I am from the spirit world; I am projected on this physical plane to fulfill a mission!"

"I am immortal; No harm can come to me!"

"I am spirit; all of nature is constantly working to heal, protect and sustain this spiritual temple that is provided for me!"

"I am spirit; No harm can come to me because I am spirit!"

"I am perfect health, eternal life, eternal youth, immaculate beauty and abundance!"

"All of Nature's abundance is mine!"

"All of Nature's abundance is mine!"

"I am enriched by the universal energy of wealth; I am one with it!"

"I am enriched by the universal energy of wealth; I am one with it!"

"I am being healed from within and without!"

"I am being healed from within and without!"

"I am wealthy, healthy, prosperous, loving, and happy!"

"I am wealthy, healthy, prosperous, loving, and happy!"

The above affirmations are for those people who have attained a level of oneness with spiritual supply, and are constantly feeling the joy of wealth.

GROUP TWO:

"I choose to be at peace with my finances and desires!"

"I choose to be at peace with my finances and desires!"

"I choose peace with mental and physical rejuvenation!"

"I choose peace with mental and physical rejuvenation!"

"I choose this day's peace with all the forces of Nature within me!"

"I choose this day's peace with all the forces of Nature within me!"

"All that the universe is producing is upon me, to express my divine nature of peace, love, beauty, tranquility, and joy!"

"All that the source provides is mine; now and always! I assimilate the riches of Heaven and I am at peace!"

You must never say "I am healthy" if you

are sick, or "I am rich" if you are experiencing the *agony* of poverty. The whole spiritual business in the manifestation of material supply is by making choices. Always start your affirmation with "I choose" or "I accept." Be sure that your conscious mind understands and accepts that whatever affirmation you choose to apply is in harmony with your understanding, conviction, and belief. Place your chosen affirmation in the most seductive places where it will intermittently attract your attention.

Whatever you consciously believe with *strong feelings*, your mind will achieve it for you. The conscious mind will not accept a lie. If your affirmation is accompanied by strong feelings, then it is true in your mind, and it shall be unto you as you believe. But if your affirmation is *not* nurtured with positive emotion that means it is a lie, because you are not experiencing the faith which is necessary to make it a *mental reality* in the mind. You must demonstrate the same degree of emotion which unpleasant experiences induce. Feeling is the substance *'emotion'* of things that you hoped for, the evidence of things that are unseen. The emotional substance which the power of belief produces is the evidence of your faith.

Spiritual supply is in the form of infinite energy. To transform that energy into things can only be accomplished by the positive use of your thought processes. When you become emotionally united in harmony with the emotional energy of a thing, that thing becomes your own in substance; you are one with it.

Should I now believe that you have intuitively journeyed back to the source that gave life to you and in preparation for your arrival has created all the abundance of this material world? Would you say that the experience is like the prodigal son on his journey back home from whence we came? This place that is home, is there not more than enough for everyone if only you receive the spirit of beauty and opulence?

Unlike the prodigal son, please visit our invisible home as often as possible to refresh the soul and enrich the spirit. As one sits in the sun to feel warm, go home to your Father's Kingdom and assimilate all the riches of his spirit and experience the true meaning of why man cannot live by bread alone. In Matthew 4:4, it is written "Man shall not live by bread alone, but by every word that proceeded out of the mouth of God."

Simple as it may seem, when diligently practiced, the above will lead you into the source of all supply. Jesus said that we should seek first the Kingdom of Heaven and its righteousness and all the things of Earth shall be added unto us. In Matthew 11:29, he says "Take my yoke (discipline) upon you, and learn of me; for I am meek and lowly in heart: and ye shall find rest unto your souls." Jesus was yoked to a way of life. He disciplined his thoughts and emotion to function in harmony with the principles of the New Testament of the Holy Bible, which his spiritual Father instructed him to teach. The understanding, practice, and teaching of those principles molded Jesus' character.

How can anyone understand Jesus' character without having the knowledge to decipher both his parables, and principles? Most of his teachings were not literal but figurative, and required one to develop a level of spiritual awareness before he or she could have understood and benefit from the lessons he taught.

He said, "My yoke is easy and my burden is light." Jesus was not stressed out with any of his needs. He relied on the source that projected him on Earth to have provided his needs, and so it was!

He understood that the source provided for the grass of the fields and the birds of the air, so why not him who is more valuable than they. You cannot develop such understanding and faith before you acquire spiritual knowledge of self, and a true relationship with the source!

He also experienced that by living in accord with the loving ways in which Nature indiscriminately distributes her abundance to the evil and good people alike with love, so too, he must forgive and pray for those who despised him. Like him we should do likewise, in order to receive divine blessing from the source. You too can find your place in the kingdom if you will adopt the ways in which nature distributes her supply. In Matthew 6: 26 Jesus appealed for our attention. "Behold the fowls of the air, for they sow not neither do they reap, nor gather into barns, yet your heavenly father feedeth them. Are ye not much better than they?"

He asked that we observe the lilies of the valley, the grass of the fields, and the birds of the air, how they receive their sustenance. Their actions express a quality that most of us have yet to understand why the source that created us and these lesser things and creatures arrayed them with such bountiful beauty and supply much so, "That not even King Solomon in all his glory was not arrayed as one of them."

Since you are not familiar with spirit and its ways and methods of supply, you therefore are not able to express the quality of dependency that the lesser creatures and things of Earth express. The only way to become acquainted is by study, practice, and understanding the psychological positive and negative ramifications of the principles that Jesus was inspired to teach. Let us examine and decipher some of them:

In John 14:6, He said "I am the way, the truth and the light, no man cometh unto the father but by me." Jesus continued to emphasize the importance of emotional discipline in almost every example he offered.

In Matthew 5:40, He warned "And if any man will sue thee at the law, and take away thy coat let him have thy cloak also." All of Jesus teaching strongly indicates the importance of emotional discipline. Study this supportive example.

Why should I give up my coat and cloak if not to prove I am not angry. Be prudent to avoid negative emotions, they are deleterious and are considered your most destructive enemies.

These principles unequivocally relate to your thought actions anytime emotions are expressed. If they are negative by nature, the persons inhibiting such thoughts and feelings shall equally pay the penalties up to the last farthing of the law according to thought principle, hence the difficulties we experience because of the actions of our individual negative emotions. The source is perfect love by nature, so we cannot be punished by the source which grants us free will of choice. In John 5:22, it is written, "For the Father judgeth no man, but hath committed all judgment unto the son." In John 5:27, "And hath given him authority to execute judgment, because he is the son of man."

Should I now believe with faith that you have understood the importance of emotional control, and why it is your greatest asset and your worst destructive enemy? Without the ability to inject emotion into your realization that you are one with the source and therefore an inheritor of the abundance of Nature's flux, your imagination shall be without life, and will not produce any result.

It is important, very important that you practice the exercise of induction to assimilate the flux of Nature's abundance daily, so that you will be constantly experiencing deep conviction of being one with spiritual supply. It is only at this level of spiritual self consciousness that you will guarantee results.

Hopefully, by now you understand that the priceless value of the above principles is revealed to ensure that you avoid the temptation of fear, hate, greed, jealousy, and deceptions. They are self-destructive in your efforts to access favorable things and conditions from the source of infinite abundance.

All emotional energies are magnetic by nature. When you are able to assimilate ethereal energies, the magnet of that emotion shall induce ebullience that will attract favorable things into your life. The law is like a two-edged sword. If you were to release energy of greed and hate to anyone it may not accomplish your wish, but surely, in time it shall make full circle and return to you with greater intensity of power; by the law of nature it shall be unto you "in kind" the same you have wished for your enemy and friends: what goes around comes around not by choice, but by a principle of divine law.

There is no escape from the penalties or

rewards, because the positive and negative ramifications of the law are built into the nature of our thought actions. When we disobey, we are brought to judgment by the principle of *our thought*. Reward and punishment are built into our spiritual nature. We are not punished by the spirit of divine love. Perfect love will not judge or punish, but we punish ourselves by the action of our own thoughts. We sin when we violate the principles of thought.

The law is divine, and we are children of the source, and inheritors of the Kingdom of Heaven; unknowingly, we are given the responsibility to bring the kingdom of heaven to Earth. We are co-creators here on Earth. Therefore it is our responsibility with help from the source to bring heaven to earth when we are so developed. Wait not for God to do it for you. It is more appropriate to say when the time comes that we will achieve adequate spiritual transformation. That which we realize in spirit shall come to pass in the flesh here on Earth. That is when the Kingdom of Heaven shall come to Earth. If you have achieved this level of spiritual conviction, I recommend the following affirmation: I am eternally young, beautiful, and rich; so shall my soul and body express.

Notepad

6

FORGIVENESS AND FAITH

When Jesus was crucified on the cross he demonstrated great tolerance, forgiveness, and faith in an invisible source. All through the crucifixion he displayed absolute discipline against negative emotion. How often he said, "Forgive them Father, for they know not what they do." That was a demonstration to us of the level of emotional control we need to develop. We have yet to achieve that degree of spiritual consciousness. Moments before Jesus took temporary leave from his body; he said, "My God, My God, why have thou forsaken me?" And subsequent to that experience of neglect by his Father, he collected his composure. His faith had been restored. Was that not proof that he conquered whatever temptation of despair that caused him to lose faith in his Heavenly Father? Here is proof that his faith had been restored as a man. He overcame the test of weakness of the flesh even on the cross. That ascertained he never lost control of his emotions.

Observe the difference of character he demonstrated previous to the crucifixion when he instructed his disciples to continue in his footsteps:

In Luke 9:3-6, "Take nothing for your journey neither staves nor script, neither bread, neither money; neither have two coats a piece. And whatsoever house ye enter into, there abide, and thence depart. And whosoever will not receive you, when ye go out of that city, shake of the very dust from your feet for a testimony *against* them." Should one forgive one's enemies but not continue to associate with them? By Jesus' example one can.

By Jesus' example, it is necessary to forgive, and love your enemies, so that you are protected from the negative forces of hate which shall detach you from the spirit of divine love. Jesus said "My brothers and sisters are those who do the will of my Father in Heaven." Cantankerous, irate persons who threaten your peace should be avoided. Nevertheless, they are worthy of your compassion.

We must pray that the spirit of wisdom visit with them, and give unto them the same measure of supply we would have for our comfort and pleasures, so that they may be transformed by the spirit of love, and become benevolent.

What degree of faith did Jesus exemplify that will transform our ways by his inspiration in believing in an invisible source? By example, like Mother Nature, he distributed all that was given to him and always received more than was required for his daily supply. He instructed his disciples to travel into distant places and teach without provision or concern for their daily requirements. He demonstrated by example, and expected them to rely on the source of life, like the lesser creatures of the Earth. He also demonstrated that his daily supply was guaranteed because of his relationship with his spiritual source.

To be conversant with the source as he was, you will have to live by the principles he taught; to ask for anything and receive it as he customarily demonstrated.

If you were to realize that everlasting life

and eternal youth had always been yours from the beginning of creation what would you do with it? Would you stay on this Earth forever? Or by association with spiritual truth, transform, become all spirit and ascend to another place by a call from someone with whom you have yet to become acquainted, if not have already known? Illumination of health, youth, and beauty is only the beginning of greater things to come. Like Jesus, we are spiritual entities of everlasting life in bodies that are also spiritual, made by our Heavenly Father.

How little do most of us know about the man Jesus? Did he not express anger when he flogged the money changers out of the temple? Was not that a demonstration of negative emotion he had expressed even though he taught and warned his congregations of the danger of anger, "Turn the other cheek, Walk an extra mile, Give up your cloak also." All of which were to have subjugated negative emotions. Did he not say that he was the son of man? And if you believeth in him, you too shall do the miracles that he performed in his Father's name, and greater things shall you do?

Jesus said, and did much to prove that he was the son of a woman but was also a child of an invisible parent.

You and I, believe it or not, are also children of that source. Like Jesus, we are inheritors.

Notepad

_____

_____

_____

_____

_____

_____

_____

_____

_____

_____

_____

_____

_____

_____

_____

_____

_____

_____

_____

7

ETERNAL YOUTH

The unlimited plethora of your share of impenetrable inheritance is there for you to access. No one can claim it. Heaven is not the place where thieves can break in and rob you of your share of the kingdom. In Matthew 6:19-20. "Lay not up for yourselves treasures upon earth, where moth and rust doeth corrupt, and where thieves break through and steal. But lay up for yourselves treasures in heaven, where neither moth nor rust doeth corrupt, and where thieves do not break through nor steal."

However, in order for you to access your

spiritual bank account in the source known to be in Heaven, you must make deposits into that account by doing well to others.

The interest in your heavenly account multiplies ten fold. The analogy of planting seeds is appropriate to illustrate our heavenly or spiritual investment. If you were to plant one corn seed, that seed will most likely produce three ears of corn. For the fun of it go to the grocery store and check the amount of seeds on one ear. That is how much your profit shall multiply in addition to your initial inheritance as a child of the source.

Since there is an inheritance for each of us in the source which projected us on this physical dimension, there must be a process through which that inheritance can be passed on to the inheritors. The thought process is the *channel* for receiving our treasures from the Kingdom and therefore must be scrupulously guarded by being obedient to the law. All you need to do in order to receive maximum protection of your invisible bank account is to be obedient to the principles and discipline of thoughts and emotion.

In order to increase your conviction as to why your body (a temple of the spirit that created the universe) must continue to rejuvenate, you must search within yourself for at least one logical reason to support this priceless truth that God's supply and you are one. Here are a few of my logical reasons: If you were to realize that you have eternal life, would you build a home, even a summer house that will last only a number of years? Or will you build one that has the capacity to withstand all unfavorable circumstances?

Since the body is designed by the perfect

spirit of love, I am convinced that a spirit of eternal life will build its temples here on Earth that is self renewable. Having realized that my body, by merits of its design, has the capacity to rejuvenate not just superficial, but every internal organ as well; the body can, and shall repair itself because of the divine principles that produce and sustains life on Earth. The body is, and shall always be a daily transitional expression of the soul's experiences.

The body is the temporary home of the soul and spirit, which by nature is immortal. So why should they live in a home that with time becomes so wizened? Every one of the creators' creation expresses such beauty. Can you think of any of his/her creation that does not express beauty? Even the pebbles on the beaches in Barbados, and the other neighboring islands express such enormous beauty. No one can deny that all the things created by nature express beauty. I challenge you to state one reason why our bodies should deteriorate and perish in death except the false illusion of aging. Having understood the principles of rejuvenation, of which I serve as an example, that these principles have transformed my life.

I assert confidently that there is no logical explanation in harmony with the principles of life, by which anyone can prove that it is natural that the body becomes sick, old, and perish in death. If sickness and death was the plan of the creator of everlasting life, Jesus would have been in violation of his Father's will, by healing the sick, and restoring life, even into his own body. Jesus' life was an illustrated teaching example of the creators will, from whom we, his children, must learn the truth of our spiritual nature, by observing Jesus' ways and following in his examples.

Because many of us believe we should get something for nothing. I shall again reiterate: Your invisible inherited profusion is *not* free! You must adapt to the principles that will bring superfluous abundance into your life before you can receive. Such discipline makes you worthy to receive the ebullience which magnet attracts plenteousness. The things you desire must first be a mental experience. It must become one with your character that will set in motion the principle of attraction (a magnetic force) to serve you. To realize you have the ability to bring imagination into material manifestation will produce indescribable joy and satisfaction.

You must personify the substance of your desire before you can have it. You must procreate the emotion "faith" of the thing which you want before you can have it. There is no other way by which you can receive spiritual wealth, other than by the principles which Jesus taught.

Notepad

8

❀

BOOKS OF THE BIBLE

The Bible is many books in one volume. It is a book of Philosophy, a book of Psychology, a book of Poetry, a book of Metaphysics, a Prayer book, a book of History and Prophecy. Some of the Bible is literal and some figurative.

Let us observe one of the psychological techniques applied by Jacob, according to Biblical history. In chapter one, a description of aging and rejuvenation as a condition of the Mind which must be treated psychologically to delete the subconscious films from whose standards we judge others on their appearances, was made.

The action of Jacob inserting white streaked rods on the edge of the water which the animals quenched their thirst was an act of psychological subconscious programming similar to the human imaginations which induce rejuvenation and meditation on becoming one with the flux of Nature's abundance. Similar actions like Jacob's is still being used today especially by business enterprises.

The following is taken from the sixth and seventh books of Moses: *"THE MAGIC OF THE ISRAELITES"*

In King James Version, you will find in Genesis 30: 37

"In the very nature of things, it is a fully established fact that the mental qualities of children differ totally from those of their parents. The fact that the sheep and the goats, upon seeing the objects which Jacob, so skillfully placed before them, brought forth their young differing in appearance from themselves has a very deep significance. Either Jacob knew what the result of this stratagem would be from appearance, or it was revealed to him in a dream, for we read in Genesis."

"And it came to pass at the time the cattle conceived, that I lifted up my eyes, and saw in a dream, and behold, the rams which leaped upon the cattle were ring streaked speckled and grizzled! With the water which they drank, and in which at the same time they saw their own reflections; they transmitted the image of the speckled rods to their young."

Acquiring knowledge to understand and achieve positive benefits by manipulation of the creative power of the subconscious phase of the Mind is not new. The above quotation describes Jacob's experiment.

Jacob placed white streaked rods at the edge of the water where the sheep and goats drank. Consequently, the streaked reflection of the white streaked rods which they saw in the water became a conscious reality in the consciousness of their mind. Subsequently they gave birth to off springs with speckled marks. Such action was indeed a psychological application of Jacob. His action is similar to the imaginations of our conscious mind that influence rejuvenation to the soul and body.

Our physiological design and functions are also designed to produce similar results of the emotional experiences of a thing or event when it is just only an idea. What was not mentioned in the quotation is the act of the sheep copulation; climax a natural supply of emotion necessary to complete the creative reproduction process.

To produce emotional experiences of a thing or event when it is just only an idea, emotion has to be induced for it is the substance that triggers the subconscious action into motion.

In the mind, methods have to be introduced to induce similar effects to those which Jacob produced with the white stakes which he positioned on the edge of the water where the animal drank. Observe that like the human mind, the other creatures on Earth are subject to similar psychological influences that can induce physical changes to their forms and features. If they were endowed with the ability to choose ideas, the ability to rejuvenate that humans are endowed with would have been also possible for them as well.

Understand that the *physiological function* of Mind and Body is the *ad-hoc*, through which Nature's beauty and opulence transcends to enrich the soul and body. As a result your magnet of spiritual fulfillment shall attract material things and conditions that express your joyful soul.

Emotion is the deciding element that brings into your life, experiences of joy or sorrow. It is therefore conclusive; consciousness that induce emotion shall manifest experiences. Not before you mentally experience (at will) a sense of oneness with the flux of Nature's supply that sustains your existence, will you gain emotional fulfillment of spiritual wealth.

To experience the joy of spiritual wealth, you must intuitively see yourself in the universality of abstract opulence. This projection of self should be practiced several times daily so that it becomes part of your self-consciousness and *another dimension of your life.* This state of awareness gives you authoritative comfort that you are in the source of abstract beauty. Hence, a prosperous future is at hand when you can feel such beauty.

Do you understand why it is mandatory that you assimilate and enrich the soul with emotional supply, in order to attract material supply by the use of affirmation; be they health, youth, beauty, peace, joy, and happiness? You must mentally become the substance of that which you desire before you can physically achieve it.

Notepad

_____

_____

_____

_____

_____

_____

_____

_____

_____

_____

_____

_____

_____

_____

_____

_____

_____

_____

_____

_____

_____

9

MEDITATION

There are many different practices of meditation recommended by several authorities on the subject such as the use of Mantra, and transcendental meditation which will produce results if your desires are for obtaining some level of peace and tranquility, but I have yet to experience any of the various forms of meditation that will produce rejuvenation of soul and body. None, but meditation, on becoming one with the flux of Mother Nature and the spirit that sets in motion what she produces. You must become one with the spiritual presence.

Jesus was very convincing with his dynamic approach and the authoritative manner in which he addressed his audience. He observed that most of the congregation was mendacious about their convictions as to how acquainted they were with God, so he expressed the obvious. The logic of the following illustrative example of God's love, his abundance, and act of giving if we apply a specific request in harmony with His principle to receive; most persons find it very difficult to understand: For this reason I must again reiterate that in Matthew 7:9-11 Jesus asked, "What man is there of you, whom if his son ask for bread, will you give him a stone? Or if he asks for a fish, will you give him a serpent? If ye then, being evil, know how to give good gifts unto your children, how much more will your Father which is in Heaven shall give good things to them that ask him?"

Jesus was not judgmental; nonetheless He did not hesitate to express observation. From Jesus' experience of God's opulence and love He was richly supplied with all that he had needed. Being acquainted with God's mercies by richly supplying our essential needs without discrimination, to all that ask of him: He suggested how they must pray: "Pray in secret, for the father who sees all things in secret shall reward you openly." Speak with your heart, not your lips, and be thankful before you receive. To demonstrate such mental attitude, your desire would have to be, in the moment, a mental reality to the soul. Such an expression of faith in God, with love for your enemies is the true and right attitude to demonstrate when you pray.

The mental attitude to refrain from envy and hate for others is the state of mind that shall induce emotion of love: that's the key to the kingdom of supply. If you have not received your request from the kingdom when you pray it means that your attitude in prayer needs to be changed.

Jesus advised that when you pray you must not use vain words for your Heavenly Father knows what you are in need of before you ask. Go into your closet and close the door behind you, and pray in secret.

"Your father in heaven who sees all things shall see and reward thee openly." This is an unequivocal description of meditation. There are several ways by which you get into meditation. The basics are as described by Jesus: You must be secretive, and quiescent. You must adjust your demeanor to a state of peacefulness. Feel inviolable because you are safe in the presence of God. Hence, no harm can come to you. That is if you begin by dispatching thoughts of love to your friends and enemies alike: This is your act of giving in meditation before you receive.

Think of the ways in which God, the spirit of love and life produces and distributes our basic needs indiscriminately. How he has arrayed the birds of the air, the lilies, and the grass with beauty and abundance. After you have entertained these thoughts for a few minutes, think of your own needs. Realize that since He gave so much to the least important creatures He will give you even more than you are capable of asking him.

POSITIVE ATTITUDE:

Decide to be nonchalant, and at peace in prayer; such should your confidence be. There is nothing that you should be concerned about because of your attitude of giving freely, loving God's creation, and knowing that God has accepted the responsibility of supplying you with all that is good and enjoyable.

When you retire from that spiritual private place within yourself or a private place such as a closet at home and still feel burdened with stress by your daily responsibilities; that will be an indication that you lack faith in the source of your supply. To doubt is to deny your rights to receive.

If your biological parent were to make you a promise, you will most likely have the assurance that they will deliver. Lay your burdens on the creator of all things; he will take care of all your needs and problems. Believe it or not he has more to give and is more reliable than a biological parent. I am likely to believe that you now have faith in the knowledge you have acquired in this book. I have been sharing this with you, so that you will achieve understanding, which should transform you into a person of dynamic character and positive energies of attraction.

As you are aware, emotion of hate will block your petition from the source of supply if your petition is of love. Your emotion of love will successfully transmit that petition to the source and you will have your request. The *subconscious phase* of your mind otherwise known as the super consciousness is not judgmental by nature; it will manifest only information that it receives.

Notepad

10

※

THE LORDS PRAYER

There is a strong advice in The Lords Prayer which reveals the necessity of emotional discipline, so let us investigate.

"Our Father which art in Heaven, Hallowed be thy name.

Thy Kingdom come. Thy will be done on earth as it is in Heaven.

Give us this day our daily bread.

And forgive us our debts, as we forgive our debtors.

And lead us not into temptation, but

deliver us from evil: For thine is the Kingdom, and the power, and the glory, for ever. AMEN"

Jesus advises that we must forgive our enemies, before we can receive God's forgiveness. In Mark 10: 25-26 Jesus warned that our Heavenly Father will not forgive our debts, if we are unable to replace the anger we feel towards our enemies with love, then our request for forgiveness shall be rejected by the subjective mind. *Forgiveness is an automatic function of the mind.*

In John 5:22 it is written, "For the Father judgeth no man, but hath committed all judgment unto the son." This means *forgiveness does not come directly from God.* But from the principles that govern our thoughts: When you are angry with your friends or enemies, it is impossible to induce emotion of love, in your petition for good things to come into the lives of your enemies from a God of perfect love, because the emotion of anger is not in harmony with thoughts of favorable gifts. Anger can only attract unfavorable things and distort your facial expression which deprives you of rejuvenation. It is obvious (from experience) that thoughts and emotion are always in harmony.

Thoughts of destruction attract emotion of hate, and thoughts of love shall induce emotion of joy and love. Therefore, you can only obtain results which are in accord with divine principles.

Emotion of *hate* will not receive approval from the Subjective Mind to pass through to the subconscious mind if the nature of the petition which it transmits is of *love*. Emotion of *love* will successfully transmit a petition whose nature is of *love*, and an emotion of anger will successfully transmit a request of destruction. The law of thought is like a two edged sword, it cuts both ways. The subconscious phase of your mind, otherwise known as the super conscious mind, is not judgmental by nature; it can only manifest and materialize the request it receives.

If the conscious mind were to dispatch a request of destruction filled with emotion of hate, the subconscious mind will adhere to that desire and supply the results. The evil spirit that produces the above negative results shall return to you as well, because you are its creator. (We create and invoke, good and evil spirits with the power of our thoughts) So you will experience the same evil that you wish for your neighbors and enemies.

When the magic of the super conscious mind, otherwise known as the genii within us is creating your destructive request, your *soul* is also experiencing that destruction as well, because the power of negative emotion which is the substance of your desire for others, makes that destructive imagination a true experience in your mind, therefore *rejuvenation* will be impossible while you think evil of others.

Such fear, anger, and hate of those thoughts that are created by your emotion become your *soul's reality* and shall subsequently manifest and distort your facial expression. So that the body in accord with the principles of divine law will manifest sickness, depression, and hate, instead of peace, joy, youth, health, love and happiness is the evidence that rejuvenation can be obtained if the thoughts are altered. That is how the principles of the thoughts work, because of the innate principles of our thoughts and emotion whereby we receive blessings or punishments.

Notepad

11

SPIRITUAL ACQUAINTANCE

You may feel challenged by your first experience in the invisible domain. Your judgment of safety, the first of any unfamiliar unexpected experience, could be challenged by surprise.

You must expect it to occur in the course of meditation. Without warning you will experience that you are in two places at the same time. That could be frightening, but there is no need to be afraid. You will become aware that you are privately at home, but experiencing things that are happening outdoors.

My first experience was shocking, because I did not have a docent. I found myself on a mountaintop and someone was walking up to reach me with arms outstretched to welcome me. The experience was not scary but shocking. I jumped out of bed and rushed to the door. My wife grabbed me by the arm, "Where are you going?" She asked. I realized it was nothing to be afraid of; it was just one of those first time experiences. I returned to bed and resumed my meditation posture and hoped that the experience would return but did not; not for that day.

You will have many such experiences. They are the evidence that you are making real progress. You can experience that you are in a rose garden, or in a recreation park, or just come face to face with a person looking at you. When you are able to communicate with people outside of your environment or in the invisible world, ask questions, and get answers, it will be like a dream; but not a dream because you will be conscious that you are awake. Be not anxious to get these experiences, they shall come unexpectedly.

At some point in this transitional growth of spiritual self-consciousness, you will have to experience that by nature of your spirit, at times you seem to be ubiquitous. Do not be confused when the experience occurs. Realize that you are a child of an omnipresent God, and it is all in the package of inheritance. Remember you are made in his/her image and likeness. Therefore, you are spirit with spiritual qualities. The experience of being in more than one place at a time is just one of them. It is a natural function with which it is necessary that you get conversant.

There is a spiritual cord that connects your physical consciousness, or should I say your body, to the soul in its travels to distant places on Earth and to other galaxies: Whenever the mind experiences total peace while in meditation, the soul enjoys temporary freedom to playfully engage in child like experiences. Such experiences you should welcome whenever they occur because subsequent to such experiences the mind is more productive because the judgmental character of your subjective phase of mind is playfully at rest.

Notepad

_____

_____

_____

_____

_____

_____

_____

_____

_____

_____

_____

_____

_____

_____

_____

_____

_____

_____

_____

_____

12

SEX AND SIN

Adam, the spirit, was perfect because he/ she was male and female in one entity. The source created Adam in his/her image and likeness, because the source of life is a spirit with both characters, male and female.

Everything that is manifested into material expression has its root in spirit. So, if the spirit of God were only male, it would have been impossible to have females on this Earth dimension.

The separation of man from his female counterpart was a spiritual experience. It was not an extraction of a rib as was told. It was Adam's desire to live in the flesh like the other creatures on Earth. Before the spiritual separation took form in Adam's mind; male from female, Adam had creative powers equal to that of our spiritual source because in that moment Adam was perfect like the source that created him male/female in one entity.

Imperfection began at the moment of that separation. God, the Father had nothing to do with it because God's perfection could not have allowed him to make an imperfect son. Initially, had God created Adam and Eve, as is now, they would *not* have been in his/her image and likeness, since God is male/female in one spirit.

It was Adam's desire and choice that caused the split between him and Eve in that period in their life; being perfect male and female in one entity, their creative powers were equal to that of the father/mother God. All Adam had to do was speak the word and the separation became flesh. It was not possible for Adam and Eve to dwell in one flesh because the male and female entity cannot be contained in the male or female temple.

Observe this analogy: When any popular entertainer performs at a concert a number of persons will faint because of the intense joy they feel. If the emotional capacity were to have doubled in one person, male/female; the body would be unable to contain both male/female emotion in one temple. Hence the reason, to live in the flesh it became necessary that they occupy separate bodies. The separation of male from female sexes caused a reduction in their individual creative emotional spirit. Hence, it is mandatory that two original soul companions be reunited as one to demonstrate that power of oneness of perfect emotional creative power. The act of the separation is in itself the fall from spiritual grace that is manifested in old age and illness.

Adam had not foreseen the unfortunate ramifications that would follow after the male/female split into separate bodies. Before the separation there was perfect harmony and love between the male/female entities which they both enjoyed in that state of spiritual perfection. To retrieve and contain the internal joy, satisfaction, and happiness which Adam enjoyed before the separation, he experimented with sex which was a temporary solution that did not last when they were in their perfect mental state called Paradise. Paradise is an innuendo for the spiritual consciousness of perfection, and they lived in the Garden of Eden which is the body, the tree being planted in the garden is the sexual reproductive organs.

At that time they both were perfect matches; man woman of the same spirit. At that time in the process of creation they both on occasion were able to enjoy the spiritual satisfaction they had before the separation, but ended when Adam and Eve began to bear children.

Are you familiar with the allegory about Cane and Abel? When Cane fell in love with Abel's spiritual mate the imperfection of this human race became a catastrophe. Adam and Eve were two rightful spiritual mates and that was fine, but when Cane took Abel's spiritual mate that was the genesis of sin. The harmony of love and creative powers that was meant to be, that Adam and Eve first enjoyed, began to diminish, in that first moment of sexual intervention between Cane and

Abel's wife.

Such mismatch between man and woman in today's society is obvious. The number of divorces between husbands and wives is astronomical. To choose a mate before you develop your spiritual self-consciousness, whereby you are able to spiritually attract your true spiritual half is the true cause of separation between husbands and wives.

It is not true that Adam should not eat of the tree of good and evil. All things which were created by God are good for the comfort and pleasure of his children. The negative applications of thoughts and lack of self-discipline produce the evils we have to endure. Could the population develop self control to refrain from sexual activities until they develop their spiritual self-consciousness? Could individuals wait and pursue sufficient understanding and acquaintance to commune his/her spiritual self, with the source of all creation (as revealed in previous chapters of this book) before he/she ventured into a sexual relationship? It is as written, seek first the kingdom of God, and his righteousness and all things shall be added unto you.

When in a state of imperfection we conceive children, they inherit our imperfection. It is common in today's society that marriages of four generations and all the siblings in a family, end in separation and divorce, because the marriages in our time do not materialize by the coming together of two spiritual forces of rightful origin attracting each other; but rather by a minister who performs the ceremony on request of the parties involved.

The experience of attracting one's spiritual mate is unlike each other. With one exception: Whenever a perfect match of the rightful Adam and Eve attract each other in an acquaintance it induces unfamiliar life energy that causes rejuvenation.

One must adequately develop spiritually to attract and acknowledge one's true spiritual mate. It will first be a mental experience while in meditation then the physical manifestation will follow. One who had such experience described it as follows:

"As in a vision, we met. She was midway between her fourteenth and fifteenth birthday. We met and she approached me with ebullience and admiration which indicated a special love. Her touch released a significant amount of energy much greater than I had experienced in the three consecutive visions I had of her in a dream state. The love she expressed in those visions was of a divine nature, greater than what I had ever experienced in any of my previous relationships. Her touch was magnetic and graceful more than I had ever experienced with any adult, and her approach was just like what had happened in one of my visions."

"Most symbolic was her eyes. When she stole glances at me, the pupil of her eyes illuminated and glow with brightness like that of the moon but with much greater intensity; so powerful that I could not continue to look into her eyes. I had to look away and steal glances to see when the brightness in her eyes would have dissipated. For it was too powerful for me to look at her face."

"Never have I ever seen such powerful glow in the eyes of a woman! Greater than the light of a full moon her eyes illuminated, because I can look at the full moon for as long as I choose. This continued to occur occasionally until the time came that I approached her to discuss what was happening between us, and how we should proceed with our friendship: It was only after that first discussion of our emotional feelings that the light has not returned. The joyful satisfaction, and happiness I experienced by just sitting with her was far greater than any love relationship I have ever shared with anyone."

Notepad

13

THE WILL OF DESTINY

We must scrutinize the ideas that gain entry into our thoughts. If they are of favorable possibilities and hope for a better future, even though unprecedented we must proceed to act on those instincts that inspire us to comply. Rejuvenation begins with spiritual obedience that induces actions of *love*. Every thought obeyed, because of love, or that conveyed the fruits of love, must be complied with innocence of an obedient child.

We cannot experience physical rejuvenation if we were to resist *ethereal ideas*, for they induce spiritual self-awareness that shall transform the soul and illuminate the body.

Is there any of us who can say that his or her actions are motivated by one's will? Many would like to believe so, but there are multitudes of evidences that prove that the decision one makes comes from a superior power; not one's will by choice.

Was it Jochebed, Moses natural mother's decision to put Moses, her loved infant in a basket on the river Nile so that his destiny would have began to unfold? Who or what inspired the Pharaoh's sister to secretly foster Moses, so that he was provided with the knowledge, power and opulence that would afford him a revered noble for the divine task which unfolded when the moment arrived for him to become God's messenger and free the Israelites from bondage?

Did Moses have insight as to how that mission would have begun? That through compassion he would murder one of the Pharaoh's subjects in defense of a slave? That through fear of his own life would flee to the desert, where God needed to have him transmuted into the mettle suitable to lead his people, the slaves, from the Pharaoh's subjugation. What power from within Moses' conscious mind commanded him to take a decision to give-up power and wealth and accept the life of a rustic shepherd? Had he known that he would marry a proletariat's daughter, become the head of a family, and subsequently be summoned by his God to return to the Pharaoh's kingdom and rescue his people?

Moses instinctively knew that his life of opulence and power must change because of the thoughts which tormented and made him depressingly unhappy;

127

in spite of his position of opulence and power in the pharaoh's kingdom.

Where is the source of power that controls our destiny by thoughts, words and deeds; having us believe it is our individual choices to fulfill its purpose and having us believe it is our freedom of choice to do so?

If you were to briefly consider the demonstration of Jesus' crucifixion. Would you agree that the moment for Judas to betray Jesus was influenced and controlled by a greater power than his own will? It was Judas' destiny to fulfill that mission of betrayal, or else how would the scriptures be fulfilled? Was he aware of it in the beginning when he became a disciple?

In this moment of understanding the inner nature of yourself, can you be sure that your actions are of your own volition? As you become acquainted with the greater power within you who makes decisions and induces ideas in your mind which you had believed to be your own; will you now willingly surrender to the glory realizing you have no choice?

All the unpleasant experiences you have had to endure were designed to have provided a spiritual degree of greater understanding of the universality of oneness within you. It is mandatory to again reiterate at this point, that the principles that govern our thoughts shall determine the kinds of teaching experiences that we as individuals shall attract, and become subjected to by subconscious choices. They are but temporary teaching experiences that shall expound our conviction of the oneness of who we are within the spiritual temple. The body is designed to transform as our consciousness of self increases or decreases accordingly.

You need to realize that we are entities of spiritual forces in a spiritual temple made of flesh, so that we may come into this state of consciousness to develop our individual knowledge of spiritual self.

That knowledge shall provide the divine individual spirit you are within, with a greater degree of spiritual self-knowledge. We all know that knowledge is power. As knowledge of self increases, power to use that knowledge also increases for the spirit within to use that consciousness of power in the spiritual dimensions; hence the purpose of the Christ on Earth to teach us the way.

At this point, I am emotionally moved to interpolate many of my personal communications with the source of the true spirit within, which is in everyone of us. If I were to comply with this emotion, I would rewrite my previous book "Wisdom

Wrapped in Experiences and Labeled Problems" (1990). Therein I described the instructions I received and demonstrated my convictions and purpose of Oneness of self. I therefore strongly recommend that you purchase a copy of it.

There are many who are afraid of criticism and of being labeled insane, if they were to reveal their personal awakened experiences of such spiritual nature. To be one of them will retard your spiritual development, when this is the most important reason that you have come into Earth's dimension.

Notepad

14

CONVICTION OF AGING IN CHILDREN

The conviction of aging is engrained at an early age in children. Many children are raised by grandparents because they are mostly at home while their parents are at work. These children acknowledge that aging is a natural process of development as a consequence of constant interaction.

"Frank," Mommy called, "Come and sit with me, I have to talk with you." "Yes, Mommy," "Frank, this is not easy for me but I have no other choice. Since Daddy died in that car accident there is never enough money to pay the bills and take care of you.

I was offered a job and cannot leave you in the house by yourself. I spoke to your grandparents and they have agreed to take care of you until my financial situation improves. We will both miss each other but it will only be for a short time I hope. Pack your things and we will leave tomorrow morning. I will stay over with you for the weekend and Monday morning I will have to leave early to be at work on time."

Saturday came and it was a very sad day for Frank. He had a sleepless night as he wondered what a bucolic life would be for him. "I will miss all my friends and have to make new ones." Frank was still in bed when his mother called, "Frank, please get out of bed; take a shower while I pack your things so that we will get an early bus."

Mom fixed the best breakfast Frank remembered ever having. As they sat to breakfast, Mom noticed how sad he was so she hugged and kissed him and said, "Do not be sad, everything will work out fine. I will come up on weekends to be with you and we will still do things together. It will only be for a while. Your grand parents love you very much, and they will take good care of you." "Yes Mommy," Frank replied as he wondered what life would be like, living with his grandparents Tom and Betty, away from his friends.

They sat on the bus, with Mom's arm around Frank's shoulder. He felt comforted. He slept through most of the journey. However, as the bus stopped at their destination, Frank awoke as the passengers were moving their bags from the storage compartment. They took a cab to granny's house. His grandparents were waiting to greet them and as they arrived they hugged and kissed. Granny cried a tear of joy, for having not seen Frank and his Mom since he was a baby.

Grand dad took Frank's suitcase and put his hands around Frank's shoulders, "Come with me young feller, we will have lots of fun together." As they walked to the house, Mom and grand ma headed for the kitchen to hold their private conversation.

Grand dad led Frank into a small bedroom and placed his suitcase on the bed, and motioned with his head, "Come," he said "Let me show you around." Behind the house there were many trees including coconut, mango, orange and fig. Grand dad and Frank proceeded on a narrow path which led to the lake about a hundred yards from the house. "Here is where I come when your Grandmother and I disagree on matters she does not understand, and in this boat I go fishing," with a cunning smile, "while she worries about my safety." Grand dad asked, "Would you like to go fishing with me sometimes?" Before Frank could reply he continued, "Well, school is still closed for summer vacation. You have another three weeks before school reopens. Would you like to go fishing tomorrow? What do you think? Shall we?" And he nodded in a way that indicates he would not accept no for an answer.

"Let us go back to the house; you see how dark those clouds are out there? I am sure supper is ready by now." As we proceed back to the house we heard voices coming towards us. He looked at me with a smile. "Do you hear that? They are coming to get us. I told you supper was ready!" Grand ma shook her head as she spoke, "Tom, could you not wait? You had to bring the child out here in this chill?" Grand dad responded, "Well, I had to get him acquainted! Do you not see the boy is having fun?" "Tom, you should know that supper would be ready by now. We should not have to come all the way down here to tell you that, while the food is getting cold on the table!" He put his hand across her shoulder and glanced at Frank. They returned to the house and headed straight to the large size kitchen table.

After supper, Frank excused himself and went into the little bedroom which was prepared for him, and noticed that Mom had already emptied his suitcase and put his clothes into the closet, but left his night clothes on his pillow. She came into the room right then, and said, "Frank, I know you should be tired. Here are your pajamas. Take a shower; and get dressed and go to bed." "Yes Mom," replied Frank. He lain in bed and thought, coming here was a good idea of Mom's after all!

Frank slept soundly all night. It was the cock crowing that woke him. Frank stayed in bed and reminisced about his previous evening's experiences when his grand mother stepped in. "Good morning Frank! Did you sleep well? I came into the room twice to check on you, but you were fast asleep. You must have been very tired?" "I usually attend the seven O'clock service every Sunday, but seeing how tired you were, I did not want to wake you. So your mother and I have agreed that the whole family would visit for the ten O'clock service."

Frank struggled out of bed and headed for the bathroom, and met his Mom in the hallway. "Good morning Frank, How did you sleep last night?" "Good, but I am still tired!" Frank exclaimed! His mother replied, "Frank, granny wants the whole family to attend the ten O'clock service with her. We must appease her request. You will have the afternoon to catch-up on your rest. After breakfast I will iron your clothes. You know granny would want to show us off to her friends."

They were all dressed up and on schedule for the Ten O'clock service. Frank had cat naps all through the service. At times it was embarrassing when he started to snore and his Mom had to jab him slightly to keep him awake. When the service concluded the family stepped out and greeted many of the parishioners in the church yard with hand shakes, hugs, and kisses. As they walked feeling refreshed with vigor granny asked, "Frank, did you enjoy the service?" Frank replied, "Granny, I did not understand one word that the minister said. What language was he speaking Granny?" "Latin," she said. "But Granny, don't you think he should

speak English so that we can all partici-
pate in the service? Can you speak Latin
Granny? "No son" Granny replied. Frank
continued, "That is why I slept through
the service!" Tom looked at Frank with a
silent grin on his face.

After lunch Frank slept all through the
evening. The following morning he dis-
appointingly realized that his mother had
left Sunday evening while he was asleep.
"Where is Mummy?" Frank asked his
grand mother. "She left yesterday while
you were asleep to get back to the City,
so that she will be on time to start work,
this Monday Morning." Frank responded, "She should have awakened me!"
Granny replied, "She kissed and wish
you well even though you were asleep."

After breakfast, Tom said to Frank, "We
will go deer hunting today because our
supply on meat is low. Tom went into one

of his bedroom closets, to fetch his rifle, and said to Frank, "When you get older I will teach you how to shoot this thing. You will have to wear a red shirt, so that no one will mistake you for a beast. Do you have such kind of gear?" "Yes, Grand dad." Frank was filled with excitement. He did not have to wait too long to see his grandfather in action. "Here comes our game," said his grand father, this is a big one!" Tom took aim and fired, "Bulls eye son, I got him. We will rest here for a while and then we will start back with our catch to the house."

They sat under a huge tree, and all was silent for a while. Then Frank asks, "Grand dad. How old are these trees?" "I do not know son, they have been here long before I was born. To me they have always been here. They express so much beauty and power." "Grand dad is it not strange that the trees can live more than a thousand years and still express so much beauty and power, but people get old, sick, and die within less than one hundred years? "If we are the children of God, why should that happen to us Grand dad?" "Son, all I know is I am sixty seven and all my bones are already aching."

"I was a sea man on a cargo ship in world war two when a German sub sank our ship. I got my knees shattered, since then, whenever, it is going to rain I can predict the showers a whole day in advance. My weather predictions are more accurate than the paid forecasters." In the same breath Grand dad said, "We should get back to the house before the rain comes." Grand dad had very strong shoulders and arms. He lifted the deer, put it across his shoulders, and held on to its legs and walked to the house without resting. Just as they got to the house it started to rain.

"Well Frank, tomorrow most likely it will rain all day, so we will stay in the house but the following day should be bright and sunny so we can go fishing." "Grand dad, I thought we will go hunting again." "No son, you go hunting two days in a row, only if you did not make a catch the first day because one catch is more than enough food for a month. You must kill only for food. You must never kill for pleasure, but you may fish every day of the week for pleasure, because you can release a fish back into the water and watch it swim away to be caught another day." Almost every day Frank and grand dad went fishing for the balance of his vacation days from school.

Notepad

_____

_____

_____

_____

_____

_____

_____

_____

_____

_____

_____

_____

_____

_____

_____

_____

_____

_____

_____

_____

15

MOTIVATION AND SELF-ESTEEM

The appropriate way to become a more successful person is to recognize that you have the ability to become more productive than you are. Not by walking in the footsteps of an idol, but by discovering that you are a special person who can achieve anything you desire. We are born with special gifts to discover and provide many special services that will enhance a better quality of life for the human race beyond our wildest dreams.

You must first awake and discover that you are a special person endowed with hidden talents that no one but you can accomplish. Many of us expend our energies trying to imitate the work of others, not realizing that we are born with hidden inherited individual gifts, and that we can give life to new ideas in service to society.

Many children are encouraged to be like an icon who have made some valuable contribution to society, not realizing that within each child there is an individual creative spirit, within whom new creation is intended to give rise to, like a seed, an idea in the mind, waiting for the spring, a time to grow and change society for the betterment of the human race.

Are you not a person of such great value? Or are you just a creature made of flesh and blood who are formed from the dust of the earth, and at the end of your days in this life, shall return to the earth from which Mother Nature has produced and sustains the physical person you are? Then, for what objective is the sustenance which Mother Nature is providing?

Realize that you are a spiritual entity within your body, whose purpose is to create from within your house of flesh, great and noble things that will give rise to the universal creative spirit who have created the Universe of beauty and opulence. You are an outer expression of that spirit.

I was in ignorance, like you, before I developed the awareness that I am a perfect spirit of God's creation, have been sent to create and express some characteristics of my spiritual self, one with the source of life whose purpose is to produce things of love and beauty that will materially express the nature and oneness with His universal spirit of creation, with whom we are one.

Once you realize that you are more than dust of the Earth, but a spirit with all the above qualities, then you can change your character by searching deep within yourself for that special gift to express that special you. However, by examples your creative ability is enslaved to the standards set forth by society.

The great majority of us, children as well as adults have allowed ourselves to be indoctrinated by society's standards which have decided for us what we must normally accept in life. Consciously and subconsciously we are given the behavioral pattern of thoughts that deprive us from excelling beyond the norms of society. When as a child the errors you make in your efforts to learn what will produce favorable results are criticized, and those actions that will produce favorable results are discouraged. Instead we are indoctrinated into accepting limited possibilities of thoughts that enslaved our creative minds and deprive us of progress.

Whenever you attempt to break free from the prison walls that limit the boundaries of your thinking you are harshly criticized and punished by parents, teachers, your siblings and peers. By doing so they consciously and sometimes subconsciously steal our life energies which they so badly need, but know no other source from which to protract that supply. They make you feel emotionally inadequate, while in the act they steal from you some of your life energies which are necessary to make them feel special. They will ignorantly feed emotional poison to your mind. They will tell you that your ideas are impossible to achieve because they themselves have already entered into arguments with society's limitations of thought possibilities. They cannot perceive the endless possibilities that are available to you. They will say that you are wasting precious time. You must fit in their limited possibilities of thoughts: finish college, get a job, get married, and survive on a limited income.

The people who discourage you from soaring above the normal expectations of society should be the ones to encourage and motivate you to pursue your dreams. They are the persons that should be teaching the children how to apply creative thinking, but they themselves know not how. So where can the young minds find instructions and encouragement as to how they must apply creative thinking? I have stated before in this book that mind teaches itself. Through the deep practice of meditation and the practice of getting into the flux of Nature's supply is the sure way of becoming an expert on creative thinking.

Every chapter in this book takes you step by step on a higher level of self-awareness which results will take you to soaring heights of self-esteem that shall inspire and motivate you to achieve remark-able discoveries never before conceive possible.

Discovering who you truly are will put you in touch with the source of positive emotional supply and provide you with *unlimited freedom from mental slavery*. From there forward you shall realize that it is only by personal efforts of mind control you can remain truly free.

Notepad

16

❦

CONVICTION OF AGING – PART TWO

Pit was very excited the first day he had to meet and get acquainted with his teachers and fellow students. Mr. Maxwell, Pit's teacher was told that Pit was a gifted basket ball player and the word went around. Pit was excited but a little nervous when Mr. Maxwell introduced him to the class.

Mr. Maxwell steps into the classroom "Good morning boys and girls we have a new student with us as of today! He is Pit Geoffrey. I heard that he is good at throwing balls into baskets. As your coach and teacher, let us welcome him into our school and basket ball team." Pit stood and acknowledged he was the new student. "Thank you Sir!" Pit replied to Mr. Maxell's introduction and invitation into the Basket Ball team.

The first break between sessions came and two boys approached him, "Hi Pit; I am Jimmy and this is Bob!" "Good to meet you, I am Pit". "Well Pit, there's always room for another student in our school, if you ever need to know anything feel free to ask, and if you like playing ball as Mr. Maxwell said; we practice three days weekly after school here at the gym. Would you like to practice with the team today?" Pit replied, "I would like to join the team but I will have to speak to my grand father this evening when I get home, and then I will stay after school and practice."

Pit returned home from school on schedule as Tom expected. "Hello Pit how was your first day at school?" "Great grand dad, it was fun. They have invited me to join the basket ball team; is that O'K with you?" "Sure, I am happy that the team has invited you to play with them." "Well, let me know when you will be scheduled to play a match so I could come to see how good a player you are. Your supper is on the kitchen table. Your grand mother is taking her regular afternoon nap so please, be quiet."

The following Sunday, the school team was scheduled to play a visiting team on the school ground, and Pit was invited to play on the team. He returned home and informed his grandfather. "Sunday we are playing against a visiting team grand dad; you are invited." "Ok son, I will be there to see you in action. I will not miss it for anything." Tom drove Pit to the games and was very proud on seeing how well Pit played. He scored the most goals for his team. It was obvious that because of Pit's performance, the home team won.

On their return drive, Pit asked his grand father "Did you enjoy the game?" "I am very proud of you son. You did very well; keep that up and you will become very famous!" His grand father replied. "Grand dad, why was there so few parents at the games?" Tom pensively considered the question before answering his grand son. "Pit, there are few jobs in our town to keep the parents at home. So, most parents live and work in distant places. Well, like us, the grandparents take care of the children while the parents live and work in other states.

The little community was made up of senior citizens, young children, and adolescents. Although Pit enjoyed the bucolic life, he missed his mother very much. "Grand dad, when did Mom say she would come to visit?" "Well son, I think she said in two weeks. Yes, that is what she said, so she should be here next weekend. It is natural to miss your mother; after all you both were attached, but you are having fun here, have you not?" "Yes, you know, I miss Mom a lot!" "Yes, I know son, but as I said, you are doing fine here; in time you will adjust."

Pit's responsibilities at home were increasing as his grand parents became less active each year and Pit gradually took over the chores of his grand father's. He learned to shoot, because he noticed that his grand father's sight had begun to fail. When they went fishing he took the oars because his grand dad was not as energetic as before, when he first came to stay with them. He had grown to love them, and decided he would not leave like the other adults.

Pit secretly decided that he accept the challenge to break this false cycle that the masses have accepted from childhood that aging is natural. He intuitively realized that every child was a subconscious victim of the aging illusion, especially the children in his community.

Pit graduated and applied for the position to replace his former teacher who was about to retire. He became the youngest teacher and basket ball coach. Pit realized how important his position was; the only young adult tutor in the school. He became the parent role model for all the students, especially for the majority of students who like himself had been raised by their grand parents. Pit could not have accepted the rapid deteriorating process of humans. He was unlike the majority that has accepted that aging was natural.

He thought to himself that in the scripture it is written, "According to thy faith, so shall it be unto you." "It seems to me that the aging process is being handed down through the centuries from generation to generation without questioning this illusion of growing old, sick, and final accepting death as natural. Jesus, the greatest of all teachers on the subject of psychology taught that sin was the cause of all manner of sickness when he said your sins have been forgiven you! Sin no more, least your infirmities shall return even worst than before.

If sin is the cause of old age, sickness and death. Then the sinless should not become old, sick, and die! Jesus used the analogy of a planter who sown seeds in the field, to describe the purpose and the expected results of his efforts as a preacher and teacher that offered new concepts as described in the New Testaments in the Holy Bible; the process of spiritual transformation.

Ignorantly, most individuals put in motion their negative emotion to create all the unpleasant experiences that they are constantly trying to solve. How much time is required for this human race to wake-up and realize this divine truth?

Even in the end of his mission, the crucifixion on the cross was a demonstration of the power and discipline he demonstrated over negative emotions! He never allowed anger to enter his thoughts, least he would have failed to prove the power of love, over sickness and death, and would not have achieved the glory of a spiritual kingdom.

I must reiterate, When Jesus took his last breath on the cross, he simply *relinquished* his body *temporarily* and thereafter returned and claim it in the tomb. Had he died on the cross, another spirit would have had to raise him from the tomb. Did he not transformed into total energy and disappear into spirit at the final stage of his mission as a teacher? That is how the creator expects us to develop on this Earth and take our departure back into the spirit world.

Jesus mission should have positively impacted the world by the examples which he lived, preached, and demonstrated those priceless treasures of the things we can accomplish, if we were to follow those principles of which he spoke. He said to one of his disciples, "Let the dead bury their dead, you who can see follow me!" If sickness and death were natural Jesus would have been in violation of the principles which he taught by healing the sick and raising the dead! Since the dead cannot bury others who are dead, then the dead he referred to were living people who were dead because they could not have understood the simple examples and illustrations of the truth he offered.

Observe how powerful the power of belief, that delude spiritual principles. One's beliefs can produce false manifestation to satisfy one that what he/she believes is true for each individual. "According to thy faith, so shall it be for you!" Each person may choose whatsoever he/she wants to believe and have it manifest in his/her life.

How few realize the priceless gift to create with one's thoughts the things one choose to believe, Mother nature actions are our protuberant paradigm but most of us continue to live in ignorance in spite of this illustrative truth.

Hence, we fit the profile that we are caught

in a wake dream of accepting all infirmities as natural, when conversely; we are individual temples of the eternal spirit of life. I urge you to wake up from your wakeful sleep and observe the truth. Like the creator we inherit everlasting life from the beginning, but most individuals put in motion the negative emotions to create all the unpleasant experiences that they constantly are trying to solve. How much time is required for this human race to wake-up and realize this divine truth?

Every action of Nature transmutes in the process of providing for our needs: The sun vaporizes water from the sea, which later condenses back to water that showers the Earth. Every action of Mother Nature which is part of the flux that produces sustenance for our existence is a demonstration that nothing completely goes out of existence but rather transforms from time to time in their service of the human race. They are our protuberant paradigm, but most of us continue to live in ignorance in spite of this illustrative truth. Hence, we fit the profile that we are caught in a wake dream of accepting all infirmities as natural, when conversely; we are individual temples of the eternal spirit of life. I urge you to wake up from your wakeful sleep and observe the truth.

When you realize that everlasting life and beauty is part of our inheritance, the body will cease to age and rejuvenation shall become natural, because *knowledge is more powerful than blind faith.* To acknowledge this truth will not only transform your body but you shall experience Heaven on Earth by just understanding this truth about your spiritual nature. This is the kind of truth that shall transform this material world to become the Kingdom of Heaven on Earth.

Notepad

_____

_____

_____

_____

_____

_____

_____

_____

_____

_____

_____

_____

_____

_____

_____

_____

_____

_____

_____

_____

17

A PRECOCIOUS CHILD

Linda was a girl only nine years of age when suddenly she began to develop some unprecedented characteristics. She was very pretty, dark skin of an African father and a mulatto mother of French and Caribbean offspring. She lived in a humble bucolic village with her parents and a brother, Lincoln, who was eleven years of age.

She became uncharacteristic, transformed into an introvert pensive child, who before had been very loquacious. Early one morning as the sun began to rise, Linda knelt on the front porch and began to chant and pray as if not conscious of anyone's presence. She pleaded with a supreme presence that sends her to Earth ignoring her disapproval. She speaks of longing to return home to a culture that none of her family recalls knowing or ever having heard of. Persons in the neighborhood began to observe the strange character Linda had become and would gossip about it.

Many such persons would scornfully laugh at Linda when they walked by as she meditated or prayed aloud. Linda became resentful of their behavior. One morning a friend of Linda's mother together with another woman (who is also a neighbor), passed on their way to work while Linda was deeply absorbed in meditation as she knelt on the front porch. 'Good morning, she greeted Linda's mother, "Why do you allow this child to behave like that? The people are talking you know!" Linda opened her eyes and looked at the woman and asked, "Are you not one of them? You talk about charities and condemn me for praying! Instead, should you not try to be a better person and stop sleeping with your friend's husband? Do you not know it is wrong to do to others what you would not want them to do to you?" The lady became very embarrassed and silently walked away in shame.

Daisy, Linda's mother, was surprised on hearing such an accusation, which had never before been heard from anyone! "Linda" she said, "You must not accuse people like that, especially my friend and neighbor." Linda responded, "Dear Mom I am very sorry to have offended you but what I said is true!" Her mother asked "who told you so?" "No one Mom, no one, I know everything about all of them!" "Linda, how can you know everything about my friends and neighbors?"

"Mommy, it is because I can hear their thoughts and know their feelings." Her mother asked, "Child, how is that possible?" Linda replied, "Mom I come from a place where it is a natural character of all people, and there we enjoy true love and friendship."

Well the secret which Linda revealed became public information, because a secret can remain secret only when it is kept between two persons. But when a third person knows about it, you know what happens. Daisy asked Linda, "Well my dear child, since you know what everyone is thinking; tell me what my thoughts are?"

Linda responded, "Mother, please do not ask me to do that, because you truly do not want me to tell what your thoughts are? "Mom if I were to reveal your thoughts you will despise me. I love you Mom, and

I want us to be friends," She emotionally embraced her mother and kissed her.

Daisy became increasingly concerned about her little girl's future: most of all about the people's increasing opinion of her child. "Promise me you will never again say such embarrassing things like that about people Linda, promise me?" Linda replied, "Mom I wish I could, but I cannot!" "Why can you not?" Her mother asks, "I do not know mom: I just cannot!"

A week afterwards, the land lord sent a carpenter to repair a broken door in the apartment. Linda's time for meditation and prayer period came. Without any concern about who was present Linda knelt a short distant away from the man, totally detach from what was going on around her. She proceeded to meditate, and thereafter, verbally said, "Dear God, forgive this friend for robbing my neighbor George and stealing his car, so that he can buy food to feed his two children Betty and Camil, lest they die of starvation, since he was out of work for so long and could not think of any other way to handle the situation; please God forgive my friend."

The carpenter looked at Linda's innocent expression of her face, packed his tools and left without any explanation as to why he was leaving. He knew that what the child said about him was true because she mentioned the names of his two daughters. Linda's brother, Lincoln, heard what his sister said about the carpenter and told their mother on her arrival home and she inquired as to the reason why the carpenter left without finishing the job. "Linda," her mother said, "Why did you say that? You are getting me in trouble with everyone around here: why Linda; why?" "Mom I saw it in my prayers. I just speak what I see!" Please Linda you have to stop that!" And Linda's response was I just have to speak what I see in my prayers, I do not know what makes me do it; it just happens."

Thereafter, Daisy became very nervous when people came around, even the relatives, or anyone passed through the yard. That went on for sometime, and Christmas day arrived. No visitors came to the house. Daisy and her two children had lunch, after which she instructed the children to shower and get dressed to take a cake she had baked for her name sake, a friend who lived a couple of miles away in another village. Daisy sat on a chair and instructed Linda to sit on the floor in front of her while she comb and platted Linda's hair in preparation for the children's journey to her friend's house.

Linda, unexpectedly said to her mother, "Mom, I am going to die! I am going back to the place I came from. People here are not ready for persons like me!" She responded, "What nonsense is this now? Sit quietly and let me comb your hair!" Linda reiterated, "Mom it is true. When I die, I want Miss Daisy to comb my hair just the way you are doing it now, because I know you will not be able to do it." Her mother replied, "I do not want to hear anymore of it! Shut your mouth so I could finish combing your hair!" So Linda said nothing more.

The two children left home on their journey to the house of their mother's friend. As they walk quietly along the edge of the road, thoughts of what his sister said to their mother occupied Lincoln's mind so he broke the silence. "Why did you say to mother you are going to die?" She replied, "It is true, I am leaving. I am going back to the place from which I came! What is not true is, people do not die because outside the body we are invisible! I am going back because I am not happy here living among people that can not appreciate people like me. I will come and visit you from time to time, I promise."

Lincoln and his sister Linda returned home that evening also with cake sent by their mother's friend and all seemed to be well until the following morning after Christmas. Linda sat on the stoop, which is a small veranda at the back of the house, nonchalantly looking at the rising Sun. Her mother found it disturbing to those who had to walk back and forth on their way to the kitchen. The kitchen was detached from the house, and was about fifteen feet away. So she said to Linda "If you do not feel well, go inside and lie in my bed, you are in the way of everyone who has to go up and down the steps."

Linda did as her mother said.

When Daisy remembered and went inside to check on her daughter; she surprisingly discovered that Linda had a very high temperature so she applied a local treatment. She mixed a drink of lime juice and honey and massaged her daughter with soft candle grease with lime juice also. From her mother's experience such treatment worked well before but not this time, because over the next three days the temperature intensified. The village doctor came to inspect Linda's condition, and he ordered that she be taken to hospital immediately. With help of her name sake friend, Daisy got both children dressed and headed to the Hospital.

When they arrived, the casualty was practically free of patients so they were sent immediately to the physician's office. The doctor examined the child and instructed the nurse and mother; "take her to the children's ward." Daisy remembered what her little girl said to her on Christmas day and as a result became increasingly scared as to what could happen. The doctor diagnosed the child to be suffering from malaria fever. Linda predicted her death, and so it came to pass, she was buried one week to date after she predicted her passing on, or it is more appropriate to say, she returned home to where she belonged. She was buried New Years day.

I remember the hymns we sang at her funeral service. The most symbolic one was, "There is a home for little children above the bright blue skies." At times, I feel her presence, even now.

This phenomenon has ever since, like many others, deeply occupied my thoughts and questions have plagued my thoughts for many years. What Linda knew at the age of eight took me sixty-two years to understand and accept. You too must accept or deny the knowledge which I have shared with you about your spiritual self. You must decide what the illusions of truth are and recognize the difference between them.

Whatsoever you choose to believe, if they attract enjoyable experiences, they shall be your blessings, but if you choose to believe in unwanted realities, they shall be your curse. Be careful what you choose to believe because you are a creator.

Notepad

18

JESUS ADOLESCENCE

Nothing is told of Jesus' teenage life in the Holy Bible. For a character of his stature, one would expect that all of his life history would have been told, so that readers would form their own judgment of the Messiah. As a child did he demonstrate the discipline of the principles he lived and taught when he became an adult?

Not many of us will attempt to challenge, even without understanding the power of truth in the principles Jesus represented, introduced, and demonstrated to the world at large. The principles which we must apply to induce rejuvenation and fullness of life are extracts from those he lived and taught. To understand rejuvenation and all it entails is an introduction to eternal life. Since there is evidential manifestation that the body can be transformed by energies of ethereal convictions, and there is no limit to such transformation which Christ demonstrated when He became total energy and ascended; was not that an act of eternal life?

It is unquestionable whether Jesus was the son of God. There is compelling evidence that he was born with special gifts and powers that exceeded all those who came before him. When as a Boy, had he the wisdom and discipline to control the power given him from birth to free the human race from sin, as written in the Bible? Was there an egoistic arrogance in Jesus' character? Allow me to challenge your judgments with the following quotes from "The Lost Books of the Bible" written by Solomon J Schepps.

"The two Gospels of Christ infancy are more problematic. In the biblical Gospel there are examples of Jesus' toughness, like his driving the money changers out of the temple, and his response to his mother at the wedding feast at Canan when he changed water into wine: "Woman, what have I to do with thee? Mine hour is not yet come" (John 2:4) but the accounts in the infancy Gospels often display Jesus with an enormous vicious ego. In The Lost Books of The Bible infancy two, for example a boy running through the streets brushes against Jesus' shoulder. Jesus in his anger causes the boy to fall down dead. When various members of the community accused him of murder, he caused them to go blind. It is not difficult to see why this piece was omitted from the Bible.

Paul is, of course, the primary interpreter of the Gospels, and all of the letters in the Bible by persons other than Paul are in thematic agreement with his letters. That is because, by the time of the Fathers - Paul's authority was so firmly entrenched that any apostolic letters differing from his own, even those without contradiction, were rejected. The three books of Harmas, for example, were recommended for use at one time or other by Jerome Origen, and Tertullian, and although these writings were never called any worst than "foolish" they were not ultimately deemed to be truly divine.

The New Testament has one main theme above all; that Christ came to save Mankind. The writings in this book are also intentionally evangelical, but they provide us with a closer look at Jesus and the world he lived in. As this period is certainly one of the most crucial in

Western history, this book should be of great interest to all."

Therein it is written that when Jesus was a baby, on many occasions, St Mary his mother gave to numerous persons who were infected with fatal diseases and others who were tormented by demonic spirits the water she washed the baby Jesus in, to sprinkle on their bodies. On doing so, their infirmities vanished, and they became whole in mind and body.

There are also historical evidences in The Lost Books of the Bible about Jesus' boyhood days, about how he demonstrated his unprecedented powers. When he was a child, many of those who displeased him he caused to drop dead.

I am not an iconoclast, but feel obligated to bring your attention to observe all the written facts of Jesus' history. As a child he got into conflicts with his peers. This also reveals that Jesus as a child did not have the discipline of emotional control that he demonstrated at the crucifixion at Calvary on the cross. At what point in his development did he achieve such discipline to be characterized: The Lamb of God who took away the sins of the world? If any of this is true; it also proves that Our Lord Jesus was not sinless: That He is a true example of the human race. With confidence, we can take on the discipline He preached, taught and demonstrated while on the cross at the crucifixion. By these examples we shall become worthy to receive all God's grace and power on Earth. Rejuvenation is accessible not by believing but by understanding the words of Jesus. We need to understand the physiological aspects of the principles of Jesus' teaching.

Notepad

19

꽃

WHY ESOTERIC?

Have you ever wondered why all the characters of the Holy Bible who were motivated to reveal their spiritual discoveries, knowledge, and understanding about spiritual truth used jargon language, parables, innuendoes, and allegories to teach a simple truth that they all thought was necessary that the public should be made aware of? Why have they kept the information secret in the process of revealing it; does it make common sense?

Why should a vital subject be esoteric, when its greatest reward can only be realized when the practice of it becomes natural to everyone? Are there secret forces in every society, throughout evolution, that have forbidden a knowledge so clearly illustrated by Mother Nature's actions which reveal some segment of it? Jesus used those natural functions of Nature to illustrate and exemplified those pungent principles he taught.

Why King David use allegories to dissemble his spiritual experiences in the twenty-third Psalm? Let us examine the obvious innuendoes by applying some paraphrasing skills. He said, "The Lord is my shepherd; I shall not want. He maketh me to lie down in green pastures."

Can you imagine King David as an animal that lie in green pastures to graze and sleep, and the Lord who is creator of all things; a shepherd? Would it not be more practical to say, The Lord is my provider, I shall not want for anything.

You have probably heard similar versions of the twenty third Psalms recited especially at funeral services on occasions. One might ask why so many versions are created by persons who felt that King David had not adequately revealed his true relationship with the creator who rewarded him favors and blessings from his source. The unanswered question is who or what prevented him from telling the unequivocal truth? The following is a complete paraphrased version of the twenty third Psalms:

The Lord is my provider I shall not want for anything.

He leads me to lie in meditation:

He takes my soul into the spirit of Peace, Love, Beauty, and abundance.

He restores my inheritance as he leads

me into the path of righteousness for the glory of His Kingdom.

Yes, though I walk in the company of people of ignorance, I will not fear evil: for you are with me; your power and grace comfort me.

You prepare a table before me in the presence of my enemies: You anoint my head with grace; my cup overflows with love.

Surely goodness and mercy shall follow me all the days of my life, so, I will dwell in the house of my lord forever.

Let us now observe Jesus' commitment and dedication against the wishes of the Church to teach the absolute truth of our spiritual nature. However so, he found it necessary to use allegories to dissemble the understanding of the subject that he was so committed to teach.

On many occasions when he induce healing to the sick: leopards, the blind, those who were tormented by demonic spirits, and even the dead he brought back to life. He said to them that received healing "Go thy way: tell no man, but show thyself to the priest." Why Jesus did instruct those who receive healing to show themselves to the priest, but not reveal it to others?

It is evident that the Church of Jesus' faith disapproved the principles which he taught and demonstrated. Why did the Church implement his crucifixion? Or, is it true that Jesus died on the cross as payment for ransom of Adam's sinful offspring?

If the crucifixion were the price paid for our sins by Jesus, why is it that there are more atrocities in the world now than before he was crucified? Or was he crucified for teaching and demonstrating the principles of *redemption* from sin?

One cannot question the love that Jesus demonstrated for his friends and followers. Because of such love and faithfulness, he accepted death, rather than refrain from teaching the knowledge that proves rejuvenation, eternal life, health, abundance, peace, joy, and happiness is a natural gift of our spiritual nature. His life on Earth was an unequivocal demonstration of all the above.

Notepad

_____

_____

_____

_____

_____

_____

_____

_____

_____

_____

_____

_____

_____

_____

_____

_____

_____

_____

_____

20

✻

UNDERSTANDING CONVERSE BELIEVERS

Among all the books which were brought together to form the Bible "The Gospel of Thomas, one of the Nag Hammadi documents, was rejected for a very different reason. It opens by saying that he who *understands* the words of Jesus will be saved. This, of course, is in *opposition* to the chosen Gospels and Paul's Epistles, which say it is he who believes, that will be saved." This quotation is taken from The Lost Books of the Bible, page 9 paragraph 3. As many who read the Bible should also read this book because the scriptures are incomplete without it.

Most of us form our opinions and beliefs on what we see rather than thoroughly analyzing the cause which produces the appearance of what we accept as true or real. We can call to mind, experiences of which the eyes have deceived us. Most of our beliefs are based on acceptance of what we see rather than attempts to understand the causes of things.

The power of understanding provides one with a "rocklike faith" because it is the result of knowledge. Whereas to put your faith on a belief based on appearance would be without merit. It is like building a house on a foundation of sand which would not survive any force which threatens its existence.

One sees aging as a natural process of life. Everyone is getting old. The body deteriorates in relation to the number of years it has lived. True, one would say; it is natural that we age and die a natural death, notwithstanding the Christ demonstration of eternal life! Aging and death is as a result of the phenomenal power of believing. *There is a degree of power in believing, because the Mind has the ability to materialize whatsoever the conscious mind believes.* But understanding the words of Jesus shall provide you with knowledge to discredit the false faith we put in believing by appearance. In this way we can be truly saved by understanding the words Jesus used, when he said *"Only Believe."*

Contrary to commanding evidence of aging, understanding the divine power of the thought process in coordination with its physiological functions (that conversely cause the body to age), are evidential proof that the body is designed to stay youthful or rejuvenate when ethereal ideas in relation to the Christ Principles are induced into the conscious mind as a result of understanding.

To stimulate your memory again, allow me to reiterate that ideas of ethereal qualities will invigorate and illuminate the conscious mind and the soul which subsequently transform the body, so that it expresses the emotion which the soul experiences as a result of divine ideas. When the masses understand this divine truth, aging and sickness will be something of the past. This cannot be attained by mere believing. It requires deep conviction by understanding the world within (the Kingdom within) which Jesus endeavored to make his congregation become aware of. Understanding the prodigious wealth of knowledge in the principles Jesus offered is the practice through which we can achieve salvation.

To rehash the subject into a spontaneous application: think of the scenario of Nature's flux for a couple of minutes; then mentally re-examine the physiological functions of the processes of thought. It is the *ad hoc* through which Nature's flux induces emotion, and how emotion is the Spiritual force that commands thoughts to take physical manifestations. Do this several times a day; and conclude that because of the above functions the body is indeed a spiritual temple for divine fulfillment of self. Also, be aware that the New Testament is a prescription for physical, mental, and spiritual well-being.

Notepad

VOCABULARIES

Abstruse
Difficult to understand.

Ad hoc
Designed for a particular purpose.

Allegories
Symbolic expression of meaning.

Assimilate
To absorb, take in; also to adapt to become.

Aver
To state positively, declare with confidence.

Bountiful
Abundant, in plentiful supply.

Bucolic
Characteristic of country life.

Congenial
Agreeable, pleasant and suitable to someone character.

Deception
The act of deceiving; fraud.

Deleterious
Harmful

Didactic
Instructive designed or intend to teach.

Dimension
Magnitude.

Dissemble
To disguise; conceal under a false appearance.

Docent
A tour guide.

Esoteric

Intended for a selected few.

Ebullience

Lively enthusiasm, high spirit.

Iconoclast

Destroyer of religious beliefs, or images.

Induction

Reasoning from particular facts; act of inducting.

Interpolate

To insert, introduce; specifically, to insert words.

Innuendo

Hint of wrong.

Inviolable

Secure from attack: secure from violence or attack.

Loquacious

Talkative.

Irate
Very angry feeling great anger.

Jargon
Language which is not used or understood by people in general.

Manifold
Numerous and varied.

Mandatory
Officially required.

Mendacious
Telling lies. False, deliberately untrue.

Mundane
Material things of the world.

Myriad
Countless, innumerable, infinite, indefinite number.

Nebulous
Unclear, hazy, vague.

Nonchalant
Calm and unconcerned about things.

Omnipresent
Present everywhere at once.

Opulence
Wealthy.

Panacea
A supposed cure for all diseases or problems.

Paradigm
A typical example of something.

Paradise
A state of being; heavenly.

Plethora
Super-abundance; excessive amount.

Profusion
Extravagant, abundance.

Pragmatic
Practical.

Precocious
Early development or maturity, especially in mental development.

Protuberant
Projecting out from the surroundings in a bulging rounded manner.

Procreate
To bring about.

Prodigious
Enormous, huge, tremendous.

Protract
To draw out, drag out.

Pungent
Caustic and pointed: expressed in or showing a witty and biting manner.

Quiescence
Be at rest, peaceful, silent become quiet.

Rejuvenate
Make young and vigorous again.

Remuneration

Just payment for work.

Replete

Richly supplied, well-stocked, filled to capacity.

Ruminate

To think carefully and at length about something.

Scenario

Plot outline; the broad picture.

Salubrious

Healthful, wholesome, or conducive to well-being.

Scrupulous

Taking pains to do something exactly right.

Subjugate

Subdue, conquer, or bring under rigid control

Subliminal
Below threshold of consciousness.

Superfluous
Being more than is necessary.

Thematic
Relating to or being a theme.

Transmute
Change from one nature to form another.

Ubiquitous
Seeming to exist everywhere at the same time.

Unequivocal
Obvious meaning; capable of

Wizened
Shriveled